Finding Your Way TO A Healthier Weight

Barbara Tanenbaum, M.A., R.D.
Junaidah Barnett, Ph.D.
Tim Cummings, M.S.W.

This work was supported by National Institutes of Health General Clinical Research Center, Grant M01RR00054.

The information contained in this book was prepared from sources which are believed to be accurate and reliable. However, the opinions expressed herein by the author do not necessarily represent the opinions or the views of the publisher. Readers are strongly advised to seek the advice of their personal health care professional(s) before proceeding with *any* changes in *any* health care program.

Canadian Cataloguing in Publication Data

Tanenbaum, Barbara, date
    Finding your way to a healthier weight

Includes bibliographical references and index.
ISBN 1–896817–06–8

    1. Weight Loss I. Barnett, Junaidah, date
II. Cummings, Tim, date III. Title.

RM222.2.T29 1998   613.2'5   C98-900382-5

Apple Publishing Company Ltd.
220 East 59th Avenue
Vancouver, British Columbia
Canada V5X 1X9
Tel (604) 214-6688 • Fax (604) 214-3566
Email: books@applepublishing.com

TABLE OF CONTENTS

Preface 1

Introduction 2

1. Before You Start 4
   Motivations for losing weight and keeping it off 4
   How much to lose 6
   How fast to lose 7
   Monitoring your weight 7
   Your past dieting experiences 8
   Associations with food from childhood 9
   Change is possible 10
   Methods to make changes 10
   Ways to make the process easier 11
   Keeping track of changes 12
   Support and non-support 13

2. Feeling Good About Yourself 15
   Self-esteem 15
   Improving self-esteem 16
   Body image 18
   Improving body image 19

3. Increasing Physical Activity 20
   Importance of physical activity 20
   Types of exercise 21
   Other considerations 23
   Overcoming resistance 24

4. Choosing Nutritious Foods 26
   A healthy diet 26
   Nutritious foods 27
   Enjoying the taste of nutritious foods 31
   Guidelines for making changes 32
   Other considerations 32
   Why eating a healthy diet makes weight
      management easier 35

5. Preventing Overeating 36
   Eat when you're hungry, stop when you're full 36
   Triggers for overeating 38
   If you do overeat 45

6. Transitioning to Long-term Weight Maintenance 47
   Adjusting to a new body weight 47
   Feelings and thoughts can sabotage
      weight maintenance 48
   Review why you gained weight in the past 50
   Monitoring your weight for maintenance 51
   Keeping up your motivation 52
   A continual learning process 53

Appendix A 56

Appendix B 57

Appendix C 59

Food Table 60

Bibliography 67

Selected References 70

Resources 71

Index 73

ACKNOWLEDGEMENTS

We are grateful to the people we interviewed for being so willing to share their weight loss and maintenance experiences for publication.

We sincerely appreciate the valuable contributions and support we received from Donna Gindes, M.S.W., Helen Hankin, M.S.W., Karen Mazzotta, R.N., Cynthia Seidman, M.S.,R.D., Patricia Stewart, Ph.D.,R.D., other colleagues, and students. The final product represents the views of the authors.

This work was carried out in the General Clinical Research Center at New England Medical Center, Boston, Massachusetts. General Clinical Research Centers are a network of approximately 80 units across the country in medical centers and academic institutions. They are supported by the National Institutes of Health and dedicated to improving the health of the public through clinical research.

PREFACE

Weight management is the ongoing process of achieving and maintaining a healthier weight. Everyone, it seems, is interested in the topic. Scientists are investigating why some people burn off fat more efficiently than others and what mechanisms control appetite. Because excess body fat increases a person's risk for health problems, health care professionals are interested in better ways to guide their patients in weight management. The public is concerned about losing weight to prevent and alleviate health problems, to feel more comfortable, and to look better.

The theme of this book is weight management for better health. People who are above a healthy weight may be more prone to medical problems such as heart disease, diabetes, high blood pressure, stroke, and certain types of cancers.

Because there can be several causes for being overweight, the path of weight loss and maintenance can be complex. Today, there are many weight loss programs available and it is often a perplexing task to make a choice. However, it is important to choose one that is appropriate for you because how you lose weight is likely to determine, in large part, whether you will be able to keep it off.

This program emphasizes making lifestyle changes in a low stress, enjoyable manner. It considers both the psychological and the physical aspects of weight management. Many of the suggestions are recommended not only to people who want to lose and maintain weight but also to anyone who wants to feel better.

INTRODUCTION

Are you thinking about losing some extra weight in a way that will be good for both your physical and emotional health? Do you want to experience the immediate reward of feeling better? And do you want to carry the feeling of good health for years to come? If you answered "yes" to these questions, then reading this book is a good place to start.

This is a guide and reference for weight management that uses four basic approaches. It presents suggestions for 1) feeling good about yourself, 2) increasing physical activity, 3) choosing nutritious foods, and 4) preventing overeating. The recommendations offered will help you make lifestyle changes in a step-by-step manner. If you wish to explore these topics further, refer to the bibliography and resources at the end. We also recommend that you see a health care professional as needed for advice about your specific needs.

The idea for this book came about because it is the mission of the General Clinical Research Center at New England Medical Center, Boston, Massachusetts (the principal teaching hospital of Tufts University School of Medicine), where the authors are affiliated, to find solutions to health problems by conducting research studies with people. Being overweight is a well-recognized health problem. We conducted a descriptive research study to gather information from people who had been through their own process of weight loss and maintenance. We developed a questionnaire based on issues we thought could affect weight management and then placed an ad in the Boston Globe and the New England Medical Center Newsletter requesting to interview people who had lost 10% or more of their body weight and maintained the weight loss for at least one year. We interviewed twenty-four people who had lost between 15 and 100 pounds and had maintained the weight loss from 1 to 10 years. You will find quotes from these people throughout the book though their real names have not been used. Some of the quotes have been edited for publication but the meaning has not been changed.

The basic structure of this book was developed from issues generally believed to affect weight management as well as from topics that surfaced in the interviews. The ideas that we have expressed arose from the people we interviewed, scientific journals, our professional experiences, and the bibliography and resources listed at the end of this book.

Some of the information in this book will be pertinent to you and some will not. *We recommend that you first skim through the book and then return to those sections that are relevant to you.* Mark off those suggestions that click with you and try to use them to make lifestyle changes. If the suggestions you have checked off are not effective, try others until you are satisfied. With time, you will come to know what works best for you.

There are questions addressed to you, the reader, throughout the book. They are designed to encourage you to stop and think about your own situation and to help you plan for the future. Answer the questions aloud to yourself or in a journal. You may also find it helpful to discuss your responses with a friend or counselor.

Please note a key concept of this weight management guide. The purpose of both the text and the quotes is to *stimulate your thinking* so that you can *adapt* the information presented to your own *unique* life. We present options but only you can decide the best course of action. We strongly agree with one person we interviewed, Anne, who wisely told us, "Everyone's experience is so individual. I'm not sure what someone else could have said to me that would have made a difference except that *you will find your own way* and I did find my own way. I think it is important that it be something you figure out yourself. That was when things started to work for me."

CHAPTER 1

BEFORE YOU START

Before you start, ask yourself what your primary motivation is for wanting to lose weight. With the guidelines presented in this chapter, map out a plan for how much to lose, how fast to lose, and how to monitor your weight loss. To help develop the best approach for yourself, draw upon past dieting experiences and your childhood associations with food. There are several methods you can use to effectively make changes. It is not easy to change old habits or establish new ones, but others have done it, and so can you.

MOTIVATIONS FOR LOSING WEIGHT AND KEEPING IT OFF

The desire for good health is a strong motivating force. Patricia tells us, "When I was overweight, I couldn't walk. I had chest pains. I was really sick." Also, Deborah had witnessed the devastating effects of cancer on her family. With commitment in her voice, she says, "I had a strong family history of breast cancer. I decided to lose weight to decrease my risk." Research studies have shown that being overweight is associated with an increased risk for heart disease, diabetes, high blood pressure, stroke, and some cancers. Weight loss can sometimes prevent or alleviate these medical problems.

Deborah was also tired of being tired and recalls, "I wanted to feel more energetic and when you are heavy, you don't have that energy." Nicole says, "I remember walking down the street extremely slowly and this older woman who was clearly in her 60's was breezing by me with her running shoes on in her little sweat suit. It just dawned on me, 'Wait a minute. Look at her. I don't have to feel this way. It's not a given. I'm doing this to myself.'"

Sometimes people want to make their lives easier in little ways and losing extra weight can have this benefit. For example, when you're overweight, sitting in seats in a movie theater can be uncomfortable and it can be frustrating to find clothes that fit. Judy remembers, "I was having trouble buying clothes. I had just turned 41 and I said, 'This is ridiculous. I should be able to buy clothes that I want at 41.'"

Be aware that some motivations for wanting to lose weight never go away, such as the desire to maintain good health and be more energetic. Other reasons are more immediate, such as wanting to look good for a special occasion like a wedding or fitting into a certain bathing suit for the summer. While such immediate goals may be effective in the short run, they are unlikely to keep you motivated for long. You'll need to establish a long-term motivation to serve you in the years to come while you strive to maintain your weight loss.

✦ *Why do you want to lose weight? Is the primary reason strong enough to motivate you to keep the weight off long-term?*

You may be motivated to begin a weight loss program but are you truly 'ready'? Being ready is difficult to define. Think back to other times in your life when you have been ready to make a significant change, such as moving to another city, changing jobs, or buying a house. Perhaps you recall a sense of determination and a willingness to invest the necessary time and energy to make that change a reality.

If you want to lose weight but unusual demands are being made on your time and energy right now, such as school, a family illness, or a job change, perhaps now is not the best time. However, you might consider making minor changes in your life to feel better. For example, you could attend an exercise class or take a meditation break during the day to relieve stress. You might be pleasantly surprised to find that weight loss is an added benefit.

✦ *Do you feel ready to begin a weight loss program?*

HOW MUCH TO LOSE

Don't lose any more weight than you believe you can keep off long-term. One way to gauge this is to lose 10 to 15 pounds at a time. After losing each 10 to 15 pounds, ask yourself if you feel confident about losing and keeping off another 10 to 15 pounds or if losing weight at this time would create stress in your life, making it more difficult to maintain the weight loss long-term. Eventually, you will want to settle at a weight at which you feel your best. For guidelines for a healthy weight, refer to *Appendix A*.

However, some people may not be able to reach a healthy weight. Patricia tells us, "I would like to get down to what a chart says I should weigh but I can't. I'm not overeating. I'm not starving myself. I can't get up any earlier to exercise. There is simply no time in the day. I have to accept this." Patricia was able to acknowledge her disappointment and accept what she wished were different. Even though you may not be able to reach your healthy weight, health does improve with each 10 to 15 pounds lost.

Be aware that it is possible to pass through the healthy weight zone into one that is clearly unhealthy. "I didn't expect to be as thin as I was at 125," recalls Anne. "My ribs stuck out, my arms were skinny. My cheeks were hollow, my collar bone stuck out. People were concerned about me. I knew 125 was too thin. I was hungry all the time, thinking about food all the time. I was really obsessing. But I liked the number, so it was tough to let it go up. But then it did go up over six months. Now I am not continuously hungry."

Nicole remembers a similar experience:"My weight management program gave a goal range. For me it was 122 to 143. Being a perfectionist, I had to aim for 122. Actually, I went below 122. I was justifying every pound because I thought someday I might be in a worse situation. But when I hit 116, I told myself I had to stop. This was almost anorexia. People told me I had lost too much weight, but I thought perhaps they were trying to sabotage me. I finally increased what I ate."

Continued weight loss can lead to serious medical problems and, if carried to the extreme, even death. If other people tell you that you are too thin, you may be below a healthy weight. Refer to the chart in *Appendix A*. If you are below a healthy weight and can't seem to eat enough food to regain the weight, seek professional help from a physician, dietitian, or social worker as soon as possible.

HOW FAST TO LOSE

Patience is a virtue, especially when trying to lose weight. Unless you have a life-threatening medical problem related to your weight, it is best to take it off slowly, at an average of one-half to one pound per week. Nicole points out, "You begin to realize that if you are going to keep it off, you will need to make some changes. Losing weight slowly gives you time to think about things and incorporate the changes into your life."

It may be less trying on your patience if you can think of shedding pounds in segments. Patricia comments, "I didn't look at 100 pounds. I said, 'I'm going to do 20 pounds at a time.' Then when it got harder, I went down to 10 pounds at a time. It's easier this way."

✦ *How do you feel about losing weight slowly?*

MONITORING YOUR WEIGHT

A reasonable way to monitor your weight is to set aside a snug fitting pair of pants to check for progressive looseness of fit. Trust that if you are making sensible step-by-step changes for weight management, your body will eventually oblige by losing the extra weight.

Although some people we interviewed did weigh themselves regularly because they felt more secure in knowing their weight, we suggest you avoid the temptation to weigh yourself daily, weekly, or monthly. Weighing yourself regularly diverts the focus away from the goal of making lifestyle changes. Also, the number on the scale can create unnecessary anxiety in your life for the following reasons:

• Bathroom scales are inaccurate. Also, if you move around on the scale, the reading changes.

• Your weight can fluctuate as much as a few pounds daily due to water retention.

• If you are doing muscle-building exercises, such as lifting weights, you may be increasing muscle mass and decreasing body fat. Because muscle weighs more than fat, the weight on the scale will not reflect this favorable change.

• The number on the scale can have a lot of power over you. As Nicole describes, "I wanted to break that dependency of the scale ruling my life. The scale would set up my day for me. Was I going to have a good mental day or a bad mental day. Was I going to give myself permission to eat if I had lost? Was I going to drive myself crazy all day and go on 600 calories that day because I had gained? My day was so linked with my body weight. I had to move on. My life has got to be more than my weight."

✦ *How do you plan to monitor your weight?*

YOUR PAST DIETING EXPERIENCES

If you're like many people, you've tried diets that you've read about in magazines or books and found these experiences unpleasant and frustrating. Joseph comments, "We've all gone on diets where we can't wait until we've lost the weight so we could go off the crazy diet!" However, if you stop to think about why dieting was difficult, you will better know what to avoid this time. Here are reasons why dieting can be difficult:

• **Physiological hunger.** Deborah learned that her downfall was real hunger. She says, "I lost a significant amount of weight on diet pills along with a 1000 calorie diet. Physiological hunger was a problem. I stayed on diet pills until I realized I was eating around them. My weight fluctuated a lot during those years." If you severely restrict what you eat, extreme hunger can make you uncomfortable, which may trigger obsessive thoughts about food that lead to overeating.

• **Feelings of deprivation.** Sarah experienced psychological as well as physiological deprivation on diets. She tells us, "I felt deprived. I would go to bed hungry. I had to beat myself on the head to keep from eating." Depriving yourself of food can feel like self-inflicted punishment, which can promote low self-esteem, a set-up for emotional overeating.

- **Foods that are not 'interesting.'** Linda recalls, "I was eating vegetables all the time, really not liking what I was eating. I would eat fattening foods, too, just to keep it interesting." Eating foods that are not perceived as 'interesting' often leads to obsessive thoughts about food and overeating.

In addition, when the body does not get enough calories, it reacts as if it were 'starving.' In order to conserve resources, the body's metabolism slows down, making it more difficult to burn off excess body fat.

✦ *What diets have you been on in the past?*
What can you learn from these experiences?

ASSOCIATIONS WITH FOOD FROM CHILDHOOD

Your family's lifestyle and beliefs about food when you were growing up may be influencing your current eating habits. However, once you become aware of how your past is affecting your present behavior, you can begin to take steps to change your eating patterns.

"My parents were in the restaurant business. My father would bring home food from the restaurant. Food was all that was talked about over dinner. It wasn't a very pleasant time. It was very anxiety ridden," recalls Nicole. As a child, she associated food with anxiety and it took her many years to relate calmly to food.

Sarah remembers, "I grew up during the Depression. There was enough food but you didn't waste it. You ate everything on your plate. We weren't allowed to eat between meals, although I do now." Before she could make progress, Sarah had to free herself from an expectation imposed by other people.

Jean also had to change beliefs that stemmed from her childhood but couldn't seem to make it happen until she improved her self-esteem. She tells us, "You don't have to eat what is put down in front of you. I think this is a carryover from when I was a kid. It took me a long time to realize this. It's my right not to finish it. I got over the guilt."

✦ *What are your associations with food from childhood?*

CHANGE IS POSSIBLE

People who are striving to improve the quality of their lives do alter their behavior to achieve their goals. Here's proof!

Anne: "Exercise really does get to be a habit. You do look forward to it and you want to do it."

Patricia: "Prior to losing weight, my lifestyle was sedentary. I was not involved in sports. I was eating a typical [high fat] American diet."

Linda: "I never could keep cookies or ice cream around the house because I felt I had to eat them. Now, I can keep whatever I want around the house."

METHODS TO MAKE CHANGES

Methods you can use to make it easier to change are briefly defined below. These methods are tools you'll need in the next four chapters entitled 'Feeling Good About Yourself,' 'Increasing Physical Activity,' 'Choosing Nutritious Foods,' and 'Preventing Overeating.'

Behavioral modification therapy

You can use this method by substituting a helpful behavior for a harmful one or by introducing a beneficial behavior.

Example: You would like to eat a wider variety of whole grains. A new behavior would be to purchase one new grain each week.

Identifying your feelings

Feelings also affect behavior. If you can identify those feelings, you will be in control and better able to change your behavior in a positive direction.

Example: Imagine that you are about to pull your car into a parking spot and another driver cuts you off. Rather than repress your feelings and overeat when you arrive home, you would acknowledge your feelings of anger to yourself or to another person and practice a stress reduction technique.

Cognitive therapy techniques

We all carry out mental conversations with ourselves. These internal discussions are referred to as 'inner voices' or 'self-talk.' Changing your thinking patterns can help change your feelings and behavior. Cognitive therapy aims to change irrational to rational thinking.

Example: Pretend that you just had an interview for a job you really want. Using cognitive therapy, you would remind yourself of all the reasons the interview went well rather than focusing on what you were unhappy about. Negative thinking lowers self-esteem and causes stress which can lead to overeating.

Affirmations

Using this method, you would state in the present tense whatever thought or behavior you would like to make a reality. The affirmation should be realistic, brief, and positive. You would repeat it several times a day. Eventually, the affirmation will seem more and more possible and you may find ways to make it a reality.

Example: If you wanted to feel good about yourself, you would say, "I'm glad to be me."

Visualization

With visualization you would picture yourself having already changed a behavior. The image should be vivid and practiced a few times a day. The visualization will seem more and more possible and you may find ways to make it a reality.

Example: If you wanted to increase your physical activity by attending an exercise class, you would visualize yourself being in that class.

WAYS TO MAKE THE PROCESS EASIER

• Be aware that you have to *want* to change before you actually can make a change.

- Do not make too many changes at one time because this can be stressful.
- Break down any change you want to make into small steps, each one being achievable.
- Realize that it usually takes several trys before you can change an established habit. Acknowledge with patience the 'learning curve.' In the beginning, you are likely to experience more failures than successes, but after a while successes will become more frequent and eventually the new habit will seem natural.
- Once you have changed a behavior, reward yourself with something other than food, like buying yourself a gift, going to a movie, taking a long walk, buying yourself flowers, or reading a novel. This reinforces your behavioral change and marks a step forward in the process of weight management.
- Practice stress management. Ways to cope with stress are listed on page 40. Making changes is easier if you are relaxed and able to think clearly.
- Realize that success in altering a behavior in one area of your life can give you confidence to make changes in other areas. If it is easier for you to learn how to change a behavior not related to weight management, succeed at this endeavor first and then apply your skills to weight management. This was Sarah's experience: "I stopped drinking coffee. I had a mood change, a steady state of feeling better, like a state of euphoria. That taught me that it was easy to make the change. It wasn't punitive and I felt better. It was instructional and I applied it to weight management."

✦ *Have you ever successfully changed a harmful behavior? If so, how?*

KEEPING TRACK OF CHANGES

Keeping a written record of your progress enables you to see patterns of harmful behavior as well as successes in making changes.

- To become more aware of your thoughts and feelings related to your self-esteem and body image, write about them in a journal. For example, you might write, "I felt that I did a terrible job on my project at work, even though everyone told me they loved what I did." Or "I felt self-conscious about the way I looked in my bathing suit at the beach today, but if I hadn't gone, I would have missed a great time!"

• To keep a record of your physical activity, write down the time of day, type of activity, and duration as well as your thoughts and feelings before and after. For example, you might write, "Went for a 30-minute walk in the evening. I felt less tired afterwards!"

• To review your eating habits, record when and where you eat as well as the kind and amount of food and any comments about your emotional state. For example, you might write, "I tried a new vegetable today and I actually enjoyed the taste!" Or "8pm—living room—watching TV—large bag popcorn—wasn't hungry, was bored." Judy has benefited from such records and comments, "It's so easy to pick at food but if I write it down, I can say, 'I really did eat a lot today.' I can rationalize a lot in my mind. Writing it down makes me face it."

SUPPORT AND NON-SUPPORT

Sometimes change is possible only with the help of a friend, counselor, dietitian, or support group. They can provide emotional support and offer ideas for problem solving. In forming your support system, you may want to try several options before you find ones you feel comfortable with.

"When I was in college, I had a friend who was struggling with her weight," Linda tells us. "Together we talked each other into watching what we ate and I think that was one of the motivating factors that brought me down to the weight I am now." Phyllis, on the other hand, enjoyed being in a group because she knew that "any problem is easier when you realize you aren't the only one who has it. It does make you feel better."

At some point your need for outside support may lessen, but you may still want to have it there 'just in case.' Diane knew the comfort of having such a group. She notes, "I went to my weight management meetings, but as soon as I felt I could handle it on my own, I stopped going regularly. If I feel that I am getting out of control and need some help, I go again."

◆ *Who is part of your support system—*
friends, relatives, counselor, support group?

Though most friends and relatives will be supportive, you can't expect everyone to encourage you. It's important to know who you can count on for support and whose advice, although given with good intentions, you do not want to take. Moreover, how you interact with those who are not supportive may make a difference in your ability to stick with your program. Here are a few examples of successful interactions:

Linda: "I feel I am different from the rest of my family. I just can't sit and eat and eat. They have accepted it. They say, 'She's not going to eat this.' My Mom will nag a bit. I will say, 'Mom, I'm not hungry,' and that will be the end of it." *Coping skill: persistence.*

Marion: "Some people, like my daughter, will say, 'Oh, Mom, you worry too much about your weight.' It probably comes across that way. The rewards of having lost weight and staying thin are enough to balance out the effort." *Coping skill: reasons that the benefits are worth the effort.*

Phyllis: "My dearest friend asked me, 'How long do you think you are going to keep this weight off?' Well, I wouldn't give her the satisfaction of saying, 'Oh, I knew you couldn't do it.'" *Coping skill: maintains self-confidence.*

◆ *Who might not support your weight loss efforts?*
How might you respond to their comments and behavior?

CHAPTER 2

FEELING GOOD ABOUT YOURSELF

Weight management is easier when you feel good about yourself. But you may have to work on improving your self-esteem and body image to get there. By realizing the origins of low self-esteem and negative body image and by applying a few techniques, you can learn to truly appreciate yourself inside and out.

SELF-ESTEEM

People with good self-esteem have feelings of self-worth, self-respect, and competency. Thoughts like these pass through their minds: "I deserve to have good things happen to me," "I want to be treated well," "I can do it," "I'm glad to be me." They value themselves and the contributions they make.

Self-esteem is basically an internal support system that helps you function well in work and social relationships. A positive self-image enables you to develop your potential. An upward spiral is created when self-esteem leads to self-confidence and appreciation for your achievements, which leads to even greater self-esteem.

On the other hand, people with low self-esteem tend to feel worthless and incompetent. They are quick to take the blame for mistakes and failures that might occur in their lives when, in reality, they are not to blame. They tend to be unnecessarily self-critical and experience nagging feelings of inferiority.

The effects of low self-esteem surface in both work and social situations. The feeling of incompetence may prevent people with low self-esteem from finding work they truly enjoy. Anticipating that no one will like them, because they do not like themselves, they have difficulty forming and holding onto satisfying social relationships.

✦ *How do you rate your self-esteem?*
Has low self-esteem affected your life?

The origins of low self-esteem is a complex topic but here we attempt to offer a few sources. For example, during childhood and adolescence, low self-esteem may come from the disparaging words and behavior of family, teachers, or friends. As an adult, it may be the result of an abusive relationship. Also, society gives negative messages that overweight people are 'lazy' and 'undisciplined.'

✦ *If you think you have low self-esteem,*
where do you think it comes from?

IMPROVING SELF-ESTEEM

Striving for improved self-esteem takes diligence but, over time, it can be improved. Here are some ways to enhance your feelings of self-worth:

• Realize that you are unique. There is no one else in the world like you.

• Make a mental note when you criticize yourself. Just being aware of how often you put yourself down may help you realize that you are your own worst critic.

• If a negative thought about yourself crosses your mind, counter it with a positive one. For example, one 'inner voice' might say, "I'm so dumb because I just can't learn languages." Another voice might say, "But learning math does come easy to me."

• Be aware of your posture. Stand and sit up tall, and you will feel better about yourself.

• Recognize when you are punishing yourself because you believe you have done something 'bad.' For example, because you forgot to call your best friend on her birthday, you feel you are unworthy of a call when your birthday comes around. But no one is perfect. Tell yourself that you are still a good person. You just don't get it 'right' all the time, but you still deserve to have good things happen to you.

- Don't be ashamed of your negative thoughts and feelings. It's okay to have them as long as you do not hurt yourself or others.

- If you find yourself in situations that are damaging to your self-esteem, make an effort to get out of them or learn how to better stand up for yourself. This may be difficult for those in abusive relationships. If you are afraid and feel trapped, seek professional guidance from a social worker, pastoral counselor, or self-help group.

- Learn assertiveness training techniques by taking courses or reading books.

- Make a list of your attributes and accomplishments. Can't do it? Think of one each week and before long, you will have a substantial list. Examples are working your way through school, being conscientious, having a lot of friends, etc.

- Learn to respect and accept yourself for who you are.

- Value what you need and want.

- Visualize yourself as a person with good self-esteem. Imagine what this person would say or do.

- When you are trying to meet a goal, do it in stages with smaller, achievable goals. In this way you set yourself up for success and gain self-confidence.

- If you make what you consider to be a 'mistake,' don't berate yourself. Instead, forgive yourself and learn from the experience so you can avoid the same pitfalls in the future.

- Treat yourself special by setting aside time and resources to do what you enjoy. For example, you want to watch a certain video. Make this a priority when planning how you spend your free time.

- Don't waste time wishing you were like someone else. This is just another way of criticizing yourself.

- Expect to be treated with respect.

• Develop your hidden talents. You may have latent artistic, musical, or writing talents. Expressing your thoughts and feelings through art is a way of discovering more about yourself.

• Treat yourself as you would a friend by being patient, kind, and compassionate.

✦ *How can you improve your self-esteem?*

How is self-esteem related to weight management? Good self-esteem makes achieving weight management easier because people who believe in themselves have a better chance of actually succeeding. Planning and maintaining an exercise program, preparing nutritious meals and snacks, and dealing with stress seem more possible. Because people with self-esteem feel they deserve the good feelings that come with weight management, they strive to capture and hold onto those feelings.

BODY IMAGE

Body image is the perception of body size and shape. For example, thighs can be seen as 'heavy' or 'thin,' stomachs as 'flat' or 'large.' Body image can be distorted. If you're like many people, you're satisfied with some parts of your body but not others.

✦ *Are you critical of parts of your body?*

The beginning of society's current problem with negative body image dates back to the 1970s. Since then, women have been bombarded with images of underweight models. Many women are striving for a 'standard' that is unhealthy. Moreover, when they are physically incapable of reaching this 'standard,' they feel frustrated and dissatisfied with their bodies and themselves.

A negative body image can also come from life experiences. From childhood, it can be the result of teasing by other children. Linda, even as an adult in her thirties, remembers the pain from childhood as she tells us, "Kids laughed at me for being overweight. Kids can be cruel to one another. That sticks in my mind." Because teenagers want to be like their friends, anyone who felt their body was different as an adolescent, may still be carrying around a negative body image that developed then. Because our society is youth-oriented, older people may feel ashamed of their body.

✦ *Where did your negative feelings about your body come from?*

IMPROVING BODY IMAGE

Here are suggestions for improving body image:

- Understand that the advertising industry has set the standards. Don't give them the power to make you critical of your own body. Jean was able to overcome these messages. She says, "I had to recognize that it was more important for me to feel good, to feel healthy, than it was to have this image that society wants us to have. I don't have thin legs but they are firm, and I have to be happy with that."

- Learn to like the parts of your body that you are unhappy with by looking in the mirror and telling yourself that you appreciate them, no matter what their size or shape. It's not easy to do this!

However, your body is more than a body image. If you respect your body, how your body looks to you will become less important. Learn to:

- Appreciate that seemingly simple movements, such as bending a finger or lifting a foot, are internally quite complex—in short, an everyday miracle!

- Become aware of how your body feels in various emotional states—happiness, depression, fear, etc.—and respect it for being so sensitive.

✦ *How can you improve your body image?*

How is a negative body image related to weight management? It feeds low self-esteem because it leads to feelings of shame, inferiority, and self-consciousness. Also, people with a negative body image can be so ashamed of their bodies that they are unlikely to enjoy or even engage in physical activity, which is key to successful weight management.

CHAPTER 3

INCREASING PHYSICAL ACTIVITY

Physical activity is important for weight management and good health. You can plan out an enjoyable program for yourself and learn how to overcome resistance to exercise.

IMPORTANCE OF PHYSICAL ACTIVITY

Physical activity can reduce risk for heart disease, diabetes, osteoporosis, and high blood pressure and boost the immune system. It can increase circulation, which makes nutrients more available to cells and allows waste products to be more readily removed from cells and the body.

Making physical activity a part of your daily life can make weight loss and maintenance much easier. Physical activity can help prevent emotional overeating by relieving stress, decreasing appetite, lessening fatigue, and improving mood. Aerobic exercise, such as brisk walking, will temporarily increase the rate at which your body burns fat. Strengthening exercises build up muscle mass, and the more muscle mass you have, the more calories you will burn.

If you still have doubts about the importance of physical activity for good health and weight management, read these affirming comments:

Sarah: "For me, exercise is very important. I feel exercise decreases my appetite and I feel a lot better."

Marion: "Exercise reduces stress. I find that if I'm not sleeping well, it might be a day when I've missed walking."

Nicole: "I realize how much exercise helps to maintain my weight and it just makes me feel good."

✦ *Which benefits of physical activity appeal to you?*

TYPES OF EXERCISE

Stretching

Stretching increases flexibility, relieves tension, and prevents fatigue.

• To learn these exercises, attend a class, watch a reputable television program, or see a physical therapist. Try stretching exercises designed for muscles of the arms, legs, back, sides, chest, and neck.

• Before stretching, warm up to increase the circulation to your muscles. Do a whole body exercise, such as walking, for five minutes. (If indoors, walk several steps forwards and backwards.)

• Stretch slowly and smoothly without bouncing. You should not feel pain. Hold the stretch for up to 30 seconds and release.

• Do not hold your breath while exercising. Breathe deeply, expanding your abdomen, to increase the oxygen supply to the cells.

• Stretch daily to increase flexibility.

Aerobics

Activities that moderately increase the heart rate and breathing are aerobic. They work the heart muscle, temporarily increase metabolism, and build muscle strength.

• If you have a pre-existing medical condition or a family history of heart disease, discuss your aerobic exercise program with your physician. Also, be cautious if you are over 40, smoke, or are more than 20% overweight.

• Warm up as you would for stretching.

• After a warm up, stretch the muscles you will be exercising to increase their flexibility. For example, if you plan to cycle, stretch out the muscles of your front and back thighs and your calves. If muscles are tight, they can be torn when vigorously exercised and can then take a long time to heal.

• Try walking as an aerobic exercise. It's something just about everyone can do. The way to walk is to roll your foot from heel to toe. Your knee should be slightly bent, not locked. Keep your head lifted upwards. The stride should be comfortable, not too broad.

• Consider other types of aerobic exercise such as swimming, low impact aerobics, cycling, dancing, jogging, tennis, and water aerobics.

• Avoid exercising the same muscle group in the same way two days in a row. Instead, work one group one day and another the next. For example, you might exercise your upper arms and back one day by using a rowing machine and give them a rest the next by cycling. Resting for a day or two gives the muscle time to repair any cellular 'damage' that has occurred which is actually the way the muscle strengthens itself. If you don't rest, you can experience muscle fatigue.

• Exercise most days of the week for at least 20 to 30 minutes.

• Do not overexert yourself. You should be able to talk comfortably during an activity. After exercising, you want to feel energized, not exhausted.

• Build up gradually. For example, you might decide to increase your physical activity by walking 10 minutes each day for the first week, increasing to 11 minutes the second week, and so forth, plateauing when you have reached a comfortable level.

• Be alert to signs of overexertion such as pain, difficulty breathing, nausea, and dizziness. If you have chest or shoulder pain, a very rapid heart rate, or an irregular heart beat, stop exercising and see a doctor as soon as possible to check out these symptoms.

• If you have muscle pain during physical activity, discontinue the activity and apply ice to the area for 20–30 minutes. If the pain is in your arm or leg, elevate the limb. Consult your physician and reevaluate your exercise program.

• When you've finished exercising, cool down by gradually decreasing the intensity over five to ten minutes until your heart rate returns to normal. This will prevent a shock to your heart. Then, stretch your muscles again.

• Drink plenty of water before, during, and after an exercise workout.

Strength Training

Having stronger muscles will enable you to function better and will increase your endurance. Also, the more muscle mass you have, the more calories your body will burn off.

When muscles are faced with resistance, they grow stronger. After a warm-up and stretching, muscles of the legs, arms, back, and chest can be strengthened with the aid of weights and a variety of other special equipment. First learn about these exercises by reading books and viewing reputable exercise videos on strength training. Then work with a trained professional such as an exercise physiologist or physical therapist to learn to do them properly. If you have health concerns, consult your physician.

✦ *How do you plan to increase your physical activity?*

OTHER CONSIDERATIONS

Choosing an activity you enjoy

After an injury, Marion admitted to herself that she did not enjoy the physical activity she had chosen. She tells us, "I used to jog. Then I broke my patella [a knee bone]. I never really liked jogging. I decided there were lots of other things I could do besides pounding the pavement." Linda knew what she liked and didn't like, and says, "I don't like structured exercise. I do enjoy walking."

Consistency

Schedule time for physical activity into each day. Try to be consistent, but be prepared for days when time is at a premium by having an alternative plan.

When

Block out the best time of day to exercise: early in the morning, at midday, in the early evening, or anytime in between, depending on your work schedule and lifestyle. Judy decided that morning was the best time. Her reasoning went like this: "I hate thinking about exercise. That's why I do it at 6 o'clock in the morning, so I don't spend the evening saying, 'I'll do it tonight. I'll do it tomorrow.'"

Where

You might want to exercise in the privacy of your home in a room that feels comfortable or you might enjoy the group atmosphere of a class at a YMCA, health club, or adult education center.

Companionship

Some people prefer to walk, jog, or cycle with another person. If you've made an appointment with someone else, you will be less likely to back out. Try to motivate a friend or family member to be your exercise partner. Other people prefer to exercise by themselves, using the time to clear their minds or to try to find a solution to a problem without distractions.

Change of season

Plan ahead for seasonal changes because activities for warm weather might not work well in the winter, when you're less likely to venture outside. For example, you might choose to walk in a shopping mall, attend a weekly exercise class, or exercise along with a video. Being less active in the winter is a common downfall.

Travel

Whenever you travel, plan to engage in some type of physical activity. Swimming in hotel pools and walking are options.

OVERCOMING RESISTANCE

You may feel like Deborah, who comments, "I have a feeling that there is a hard core group of us out there who are not going to enjoy exercise." Our bodies are not meant to be sedentary. With some thought, you can learn to overcome your resistance.

First, determine if you are making excuses. Here are a few examples of common excuses: "I don't have time," "I feel tired," "It's too cold outside."

✦ *Do you make excuses?*

Although you know that exercise is healthy for you, you may need to gently encourage yourself. Here are some ways to overcome your resistance to exercise:

- Set realistic goals that you can accomplish and feel good about. Otherwise, you may avoid physical activity because you are afraid of 'failing.'

- For meeting your goals, plan to reward yourself in ways not related to food, such as buying yourself a present or taking time to relax.

- If you have pain when exercising, see a physical therapist to learn therapeutic exercises.

- Wear comfortable clothing and shoes that provide proper support.

- If you believe that an experience from your past is getting in the way, acknowledge this to yourself and move forward.

- Resist comparing your body to others and wishing you were thinner. This type of thinking generates shame and creates an unnecessary obstacle to exercise.

- Recall the benefits of physical activity.

- Periodically review your exercise program. If there have been changes in your life, you may need to adjust your program accordingly.

- Write down your thoughts and feelings about why you lack motivation.

- Set a timer for five (or more) minutes and tell yourself that this is your exercise time. This will cut down on any distractions.

- If you find exercising boring, listen to a radio or watch television. Plan a variety of physical activities.

- Visualize yourself really being absorbed in physical activity.

- To help develop a positive attitude, use affirmations, such as "I like to exercise."

- Think of others you know who exercise and derive inspiration from them, thinking, "If they can do it, so can I."

- Remember Judy's words: "Afterwards, I really do feel good. Sometimes, I'm halfway through working out on the treadmill and I think, 'This isn't so bad.'"

✦ *How can you overcome your resistance to exercise?*

CHAPTER 4

CHOOSING NUTRITIOUS FOODS

In addition to physical activity, a healthy diet is important for weight management and good health. Learn to thoughtfully choose and to enjoy the food you eat. Weight management is easier if you eat nutritious foods that also taste good.

A HEALTHY DIET

If you were to look up the word 'diet' in a medical dictionary, you might find a definition similar to this one: "Food and drink considered with regard to their nutritional qualities, composition, and effects on health."[1] This is a good definition to keep in mind as you learn to plan your healthy diet. A 'healthy' diet is one that supplies the nutrients you need to minimize your risk for disease and also help you function at your best.

The major nutrients in food are protein, carbohydrate, and fat. The body burns up carbohydrate and fat to provide you with energy, which is measured in calories. Protein is the major structural substance of cells. Other major components of food are fiber and water. Nutrients that are present in smaller quantities are minerals and vitamins, which you need to maintain bone strength and help carry out the many biochemical processes that take place in your body.

---

[1] *Mosby's Medical, Nursing & Allied Health Dictionary*, The C.V. Mosby Company, St. Louis,

In addition, plant foods such as vegetables, fruits, whole grains,[2] and legumes contain substances known as phytochemicals (phyto- means plant). Research has shown that phytochemicals have anti-cancer and anti-heart disease effects.

Because vitamins, minerals, and phytochemicals are distributed in varying amounts in different foods, it is important to eat a variety of vegetables, fruits, whole grains, and legumes. For example, instead of eating either broccoli or carrots for lunch every day, you might expand your choices to include butternut squash, kale, and brussel sprouts.

NUTRITIOUS FOODS

Below are lists of some nutritious foods organized according to the major component(s) they provide: protein, carbohydrate, fat, and/or fiber. (For grams of nutrients per portion size, refer to the *Food Table* on page 60)

SOURCES OF PROTEIN

Meats	Dairy (Reduced Fat)	Legumes	Other
beef (lean)	cottage cheese	adzuki beans	soy milk
chicken (no skin)	milk	black beans	tofu
turkey	ricotta cheese	brown beans	
egg, egg substitute	yogurt	chickpeas	
cod		kidney beans	
flounder		lentils, red, green	
haddock		lima beans	
halibut		navy beans	
salmon		pinto beans	
sole			
tuna			

Other sources of protein: Grains and vegetables also contain some protein. When you eat several portions, they contribute a significant amount of protein to the diet.

[2] Grains are the seeds of cereal grasses. Whole grains, such as brown rice, still have their nutritious outer layers (the bran and germ) intact whereas processed grains, such as white rice, lose these layers during the milling process.

A few words about beans: Beans should be stored in tightly covered jars to retard loss of flavor. Prior to cooking, rinse the beans well. Certain beans, such as lentils, cook in a relatively short time while others, such as chickpeas, take much longer. Soaking beans in water prior to cooking, and discarding this water, will decrease the cooking time. Refer to a cookbook for the amount of water you will need to cook the beans and approximate cooking times. Cooked beans can be stored in the refrigerator for two to three days.

A few words about tofu: Tofu, which is soybean curd, comes in soft and firm consistencies. It can be stored in the refrigerator for three to four days in water that is changed daily. Tofu can be baked or stewed. When cooked with other foods and sauces, it picks up those flavors. Refer to cookbooks and magazines for recipes.

SOURCES OF CARBOHYDRATE

Whole Grains and products	Fruits	Legumes	Starchy Vegetables
barley, whole	apple	adzuki beans	corn
bread, whole wheat	apricot	black beans	peas
buckwheat	banana	brown beans	potato
bulgur	blackberries	chickpeas	sweet potato
cereal, whole wheat	blueberries	kidney beans	yam
couscous, whole wheat	cantaloupe	lentils, red, green	
millet	cherries	lima beans	
oats	cranberries	navy beans	
pasta, whole wheat	dates	pinto beans	
rice, brown	figs		
wheat berries	grapefruit		
	grapes		
	nectarine, orange		
	peach		
	pear		
	plum		
	pineapple		
	prunes, raisins		
	raspberries		
	strawberries		

A few words about whole grains: Store whole grains in tightly covered jars to retard loss of flavor. Prior to cooking, rinse the grains well. A rule-of-thumb when cooking grains is to add one part grain to two parts boiling water. Cover the pot and simmer until the water is absorbed.

SOURCES OF FAT

Oils	*Nuts*	*Seeds*	*Other*
canola	almond butter	pumpkin	avocado
corn	almonds	sesame butter	mayonnaise
olive	cashew butter	(tahini)	mayonnaise, light
peanut	cashews	sesame	olives
safflower	macadamia	sunflower	peanuts
sesame	pecans		peanut butter
walnuts			

A few words about oils: Oils deteriorate when exposed to light, heat, and air. To delay this deterioration, store them in tightly closed glass bottles or jars in the refrigerator. Oils high in monounsaturated fat, such as olive and canola oil, are more stable than oils high in polyunsaturated fat, such as corn and safflower oil. Unrefined oils, available in health food stores, are recommended rather than highly processed refined oils. A recommended storage time for polyunsaturated oils is up to three months in the refrigerator.

A few words about nuts and seeds: Nuts and seeds in the shell are more stable than those already shelled. A recommended storage time for shelled nuts and seeds and for nut butters is up to three months in the refrigerator.

SOURCES OF FIBER

Vegetables	Fruits	Whole Grains (and products)	Legumes
acorn squash	apple	barley, whole	adzuki beans
alfalfa sprouts	apricot	bread, whole wheat	black beans
asparagus	banana	buckwheat	brown beans
bean sprouts	blackberries	bulgur	chickpeas
beets	blueberries	cereal, whole wheat	kidney beans
broccoli	cantaloupe	couscous,whole wheat	lentils, red, green
brussel sprouts	cherries	millet	lima beans
butternut squash	cranberries	oats	navy beans
cabbage	dates	pasta,whole wheat	pinto beans
carrots	figs	rice, brown	
cauliflower	grapefruit	wheat berries	
corn	grapes		
celery	nectarine		
collards	orange		
eggplant	peach		
green beans	pear		
greens	plum		
(dark,mixed)	pineapple		
kale	prunes		
mushrooms	raisins		
onion	raspberries		
peas	strawberries		
pepper	rhubarb		
pumpkin			
spinach			
squash, summer			
squash, winter			
string beans			
tomato			
turnip			

✦ *Which of these nutritious foods appeal to you most?*

ENJOYING THE TASTE OF NUTRITIOUS FOODS

If you are used to eating foods high in fat, sugar, and salt, you may not at first enjoy the natural tastes of nutritious foods and flavorings, but give it time. Here are suggestions to enhance your healthy eating experience:

• Add herbs and spices to vegetables, grains, beans, and tofu. Common ones are thyme, cinnamon, basil, rosemary, sage, oregano, parsley, garlic, ginger, dill, chives, onion, turmeric, cumin, and coriander. Refer to cookbooks for ideas on how to best use them. Many go well with more than one type of food, so have fun experimenting. Store them in tightly covered glass jars to retard loss of flavor and aroma.

• Mix foods together for variety. For example, combine grains with beans, grains with vegetables, and beans with vegetables. Also, you can mix two or three vegetables together for a vegetable combo dish.

• Add oils with flavor, such as olive or sesame oil, to foods. Flavor vegetables and grains with ground nuts. But remember, any oils or nuts you add to meals should be measured and eaten sparingly.

• Try tasty low fat sauces. Check out health food stores and ethnic groceries for unusual varieties. Also, prepare your own using a recipe or create your own. Tomato sauce and yogurt with herbs and spices are examples of quick, tasty sauces.

• Use a variety of cooking techniques, such as baking, steaming, broiling, stir-frying, water sautéing, and pressure cooking. Food tastes slightly different with a different cooking technique.

In addition

• Eat slowly to savor the taste and texture of food. Sarah says, "By paying attention to taste and texture, you can enjoy everything as you eat it."

• Try to be calm at mealtimes. Eating in a pleasant environment can help you relax.

• Be aware of the aroma of the food you are eating.

• View food as a way to nurture and energize yourself and it will taste better!

GUIDELINES FOR MAKING CHANGES

Food is a highly charged issue that carries many personal and cultural connotations so altering what you eat may not be easy. At a practical level, making changes means new patterns of shopping, storing food, and preparing meals. But new patterns eventually become as comfortable as old ones. It may take several weeks or even months to adapt to healthy preparations of vegetables, whole grains, and beans and to enjoy the new tastes of these nutritious foods.

To prevent yourself from becoming overwhelmed with too many changes at once, try making only one change a week. Here are some goals and specific ways to reach them:

- **Increase the amount of vegetables you eat to 3–5 servings per day.** Increase the servings of vegetables you eat at lunch and dinner. If you have one-half cup now, increase this to three-quarters or one cup. Take fresh vegetables, such as carrots and green beans, for snacks.

- **Increase the fruit you eat to 2–4 servings per day.** Take a piece of fruit as a snack instead of a high sugar, high fat dessert for lunch or dinner.

- **Replace processed grains with whole grains.** Instead of white rice, have a whole grain. Replace a high sugar, high fat snack with a whole grain snack such as one listed on pages 37 and 38.

- **Eat fewer animal sources of protein and more beans and tofu.** Plan to substitute beans or tofu for at least one meat, chicken, or fish meal each day.

- **Try new flavorings.** Experiment with a new spice or sauce.

OTHER CONSIDERATIONS

Fat in the diet

Eating too much fat will increase your risk for heart disease as well as some cancers and make losing weight more difficult. If you eat too little fat, you may feel that you are depriving yourself which could make you prone to overeating. Gradually reduce the amount of fat you eat to a comfortable level so you don't feel deprived. To improve health, the *'Dietary Guidelines for Americans,'* which are addressed to the general population, recommends that 30% or less of the total calories in the diet come from fat. Some people on healthy diets follow a 20% fat diet. For an explanation of a 20% and a 30% fat diet, refer to *Appendix B.*

Fats added to food, such as oils, nuts, and seeds, should be measured and added sparingly. Other ways to cut back on excess fat are to avoid fried foods, broil meat to drain the fat, and skim the fat from the top of soups and stews.

Diets high in saturated fat have been associated with an increased risk for heart disease, so avoid foods that are high in saturated fat such as red meat, whole milk, cream, butter, and cheese. Also, avoid 'partially hydrogenated' fat, which is found in most margarines and packaged baked goods.

Drink enough water

If you drink enough water, your cells will be well-hydrated and you will feel better. Also, fiber in the intestines combines with water to eliminate waste from the body. In addition, drinking plenty of water will help flush out waste products from the bloodstream.

The amount of water a person needs depends on body size and activity level. But a general guideline is 6–8 eight-ounce cups per day. Be sure to replenish water after exercise because more water is lost through perspiration than you might think.

If you find plain water unappealing try flavoring it with fruit juice. Rather than drinking one cup at a time, drink smaller amounts throughout the day.

Caffeine, found in coffee, soda, and tea, is a diuretic, causing water to be lost from the body. Try to cut back on caffeine gradually by substituting water, flavored water, fruit juice, decaffeinated tea, or decaffeinated coffee for caffeine-containing beverages.

Distribution of each of the major nutrients— protein, carbohydrate, fat, and fiber—among three meals

Try not to eat too much or too little at any meal. Using carbohydrate as an example, instead of having one serving of a carbohydrate food source for breakfast, one for lunch, and four for dinner, have two at each meal.

Guidelines for meal planning that would work well for most people are the following: for breakfast, a food source of protein, whole grains, and fruit; for lunch and dinner, a food source of protein, whole grains, and vegetables. For examples, refer to *Appendix C.* If you need help planning your meals, see a registered dietitian. For a referral, call your local health clinic or the American Dietetic Association Consumer Hotline at 1-800-366-1655.

After you eat, be sensitive to your energy level, clarity of thinking, and mood. Vary the types of food, the amount, and the timing of meals and snacks and eat according to what gives you a true sense of well-being. It will take time to develop this sensitivity.

Food shopping

Another key to success is having a variety of nutritious foods in the house readily available for when you are hungry. Marilyn, an organized person, tells us, "If you are hungry, a bag of chips is the easiest thing to grab, but if you have fruit in the house, that's just as easy." Schedule shopping time and bring a list of nutritious foods to purchase. Also, eat a snack before you go shopping so you won't be hungry and tempted to buy foods high in sugar and fat.

A healthy diet is affordable. The lower cost of whole grains and beans balances out the higher cost of fruits and vegetables. You will be buying less soda, chips, pastries, cookies, and ice cream, which are relatively expensive. Herbs and spices can be purchased in bulk to cut back on cost.

Preparing meals

Preparing healthy meals takes more time than eating haphazardly. To reduce the stress of food preparation:

- Develop an efficient system for preparing meals. Prepare extra food and freeze leftover portions for future meals.

- Use frozen vegetables.

- Ask other members of your household to help.

- For convenience, purchase canned beans. Canned soups with beans make a quick meal. Burritos are a tasty way to eat beans and can also be frozen for future meals.

- If you need a break from preparing meals, try healthy frozen dinners or purchase take-out salads.

- View cooking as an opportunity to be creative by trying new foods, flavorings, and methods of cooking. Phyllis proudly says, "I have become a gourmet cook within the parameters of healthy eating."

WHY EATING A HEALTHY DIET MAKES WEIGHT MANAGEMENT EASIER

You tend to eat less food when you eat a healthy diet because:

- **It is filling.** The fiber and water of vegetables, fruit, whole grains, and legumes create bulk.

- **It takes time to eat.** Because it takes longer to chew food with bulk, the part of your brain that controls appetite has more time to receive signals from your stomach that you have eaten and are no longer hungry.

- **It is tasty.** Nutritious foods and flavorings can be combined in countless, interesting ways. If you focus on and enjoy the taste of these foods at meals and snacks, you will think less about eating at other times.

CHAPTER 5

PREVENTING OVEREATING

Being able to identify when you're truly hungry and when you've had enough is an important part of weight management. A critical part of this is identifying the triggers that make you overeat. You can learn to overcome overeating.

EAT WHEN YOU'RE HUNGRY, STOP WHEN YOU'RE FULL

Eating when you're truly hungry is a source of pleasure. However, eating when you're not hungry leads to overeating, which can cause discomfort in the short-term and unwelcome weight gain in the long-term.

The first step to prevent overeating is recognizing the feeling of true hunger. This is how Linda knows when she is hungry: "My stomach grumbles and gnaws. I get light-headed and irritable." It is a good idea to eat at the first signs of real hunger because if you wait until you are too hungry, you might overeat.

✦ *Can you identify your true hunger?*

The next step is being sensitive to the feeling of having enough. This feeling of fullness precedes feeling overly full, which is easier to describe. Linda tells us, "Overly full is feeling uncomfortable, lethargic." Judy adds, "Feeling overly full is like feeling bloated."

The feeling of having your hunger satisfied without eating too much is more enjoyable than the feeling of being overly full. When you become aware of the difference, you will want to avoid overeating. This was Linda's experience: "I don't like being stuffed. I don't enjoy those big meals anymore. I'd rather eat more frequently but smaller amounts." Phyllis says, "Before, when I went out to dinner, I enjoyed everything I ate, but I felt that if you took a pin and stuck me, I would probably burst. I don't feel that way anymore when I get up from a meal, and it's a much better way to feel."

✦ *Can you describe how you feel when you are full? overly full?*

If you usually become hungry between meals, plan to have snacks mid-morning, mid-afternoon, and mid-evening. This was important to Judy, who comments, "I learned from my weight management program that eating six times a day makes sense for me."

Below are some ideas for snack foods. Portion sizes are included as a guide but not meant to be restrictive. You may need to wait 20 to 30 minutes after eating to feel relief from symptoms of physiological hunger.

SINGLE FOODS

1 piece of fruit
1/2 cup of fruit juice
1/4 cup of dried fruit
1 cup of low fat yogurt
1 cup of low fat chocolate milk
2 cups of popcorn
1 frozen juice bar
1 slice of angel food cake
2 graham crackers
1/2 cup of three bean salad
1 small whole grain muffin
1/4 cup of granola
1 cup of spoon size shredded wheat
1/2 sweet potato or yam with the skin

TWO OR MORE FOODS COMBINED

1 oz. of ready-to-eat whole wheat cereal and 4 oz. of low fat milk
1/2 baked potato with 1/2 cup of vegetables
1/2 cup brown rice with 1/2 cup of vegetables and 1 tsp. of olive oil
1 small whole wheat pita bread with 1 oz. low fat cheese and tomato
1/2 whole wheat bagel with cottage cheese
1 cup of soup with a whole grain or vegetables
1/2 cup raw vegetables with a low fat dip
1 small pita bread with 2 tablespoons avocado
1 slice of whole wheat bread with one of the following:
    1 teaspoon peanut butter, 1 ounce of tuna fish with 1 teaspoon of
    mayonnaise, 1/4 cup of low fat cottage cheese, 2 tablespoons of
    hummus, 2 teaspoons of honey, 1 tablespoon of apple butter, 2 tea-
    spoons of blackstrap molasses, 2 teaspoons of low sugar fruit preserves,
    1 teaspoon of almond butter, 1 teaspoon of peanut butter with a few
    slices of banana.

✦ *Which snacks appeal to you?*

TRIGGERS FOR OVEREATING

Overeating can range from mild to severe. Severe overeating is binge eating, which Deborah defines as "eating anything that you have in the house and not stopping until you are so full that you feel sick." Be aware of the following common triggers for overeating and methods to cope:

Emotions

Sadness, anger, loneliness, shame, guilt, fear, and frustration are emotions that actually feel physically uncomfortable. Some people have a tendency to overeat in order to numb these feelings. Here are ways to handle these emotions:

• Be aware that you are eating for emotional reasons. This may be enough to help you stop yourself from overeating.

• Talk to a friend or write in a journal about these feelings.

Thoughts

Your thoughts can make you anxious but you can replace them with calming images or thoughts.

• If thoughts are non-productively racing through your mind, practice the technique of 'thought stopping.' Switch your thinking to a relaxing image, such as being at the beach or in the woods. If the provoking thoughts return, say something positive to yourself like, "I can handle it."

• Try to avoid irrational thinking. Common types of irrational thinking are making assumptions and thinking the worst will happen.

Stress

Nicole comments, "People are always going to have stress of one kind or another in their lives, so you have to learn to deal with it in ways other than eating." You can't control what is causing you to feel stressed but you can control the way you react to it.

• Be aware of the signs of stress, such as impatience, anger, tension, headaches, tightness in the neck and shoulders, and difficulty sleeping.

• Practice relaxation techniques, such as breathing deeply by expanding your abdomen, clenching and relaxing muscles, and meditating. Learn these and other techniques by attending classes or reading books.

• Notice how your mind and body feel when you are stressed. Try to relax before you become too tense.

• Write about what is making you feel stressed.

• To relieve tension, do stretching exercises or engage in physical activity.

• Call a friend to chat.

• Don't overload your schedule, and prioritize the things that must get done.

• Get enough sleep.

• Listen to relaxing music or take a warm bath.

• Remind yourself of all the good things in your life.

- If there's a major life decision to be made or a problem that needs to be solved, tackle it in a logical manner. Get as much information as you can. Don't deny certain facts or blow others out of proportion. Then proceed to think a problem through for pros and cons of options, getting help when necessary.

- Make your home and work environments as peaceful as possible.

Fatigue

Judy tells us, "When I'm tired, I may lose control more and say, 'Oh, I want to eat this only because I'm tired, so I don't really want it.'" To prevent fatigue, try the following:

- Curtail your activities so that you do not get overtired.

- If you are tired during the day, rest by taking a 20 to 30 minute nap. If that's not possible, practice relaxation techniques.

- To improve your sleep, go to bed and get up at about the same time each day. Avoid eating or doing aerobic exercise for a few hours before you go to bed. Allow yourself time to wind down before you call it a day. Try to get seven to eight hours of sleep.

Boredom

Sarah comments, "If you are busy doing things, you aren't so busy stuffing food in." Prepare for periods of unstructured time by making a list of worthwhile and enjoyable activities to enrich your life. Rather than eating out of boredom, Nicole prefers the feeling of accomplishment: "It's good to have an exercise video at home or some little project that you have been putting off for a long time. You'll feel so much better after you've done it."

Procrastination

Going to the refrigerator may be easier than doing something you do not want to do. Sit down and think about why you are procrastinating. Do something else for a while and come back to the task later. To help yourself get started, listen to music.

'Forbidden' foods

If you tell yourself certain foods are forbidden, that makes them all the more appealing and you will probably eat more of them. Instead, give yourself permission to eat all foods. The anxiety associated with these food may dissipate.

Feeling overburdened from nurturing others

Women who feel overburdened with the responsibility of nurturing others may turn to food to nurture themselves. Eating well is a way of taking care of yourself but overeating will not make you feel good. Ask for help from family members in preparing meals and figure out short-cuts.

Using food as a reward

Some people use food to reward themselves for working hard. However, there are other ways to thank yourself that don't involve food. It can be something you enjoy doing but do not usually allow yourself the time or resources.

Food cravings

Foods high in sugar, fat, and salt are usually the object of cravings. There may be other foods that people crave because of associations from the past. Linda says, "For me, there are certain comfort foods, like rice pudding and bread. They have the connotation of home." Here are ways to take control over food cravings:

- If you crave a food high in sugar, eat whole foods that are naturally sweet-tasting, such as sweet potatoes, dried fruit, and brown rice.

- To overcome salt cravings, gradually cut back on the salt you eat. Your taste buds will eventually perceive salty foods as being 'too salty.'

- Brush your teeth for a feeling of freshness.

- Try sour-tasting foods, such as lemon juice in water and grapefruit juice, or spicy foods, such as whole grains and vegetables with spices added.

- Breathe deeply by expanding your abdomen and slowly to relax until the craving passes.

- Try to avoid seeing and smelling foods that could trigger food cravings. Store foods that you typically crave on a top shelf or out of sight in a brown paper bag. If possible, don't keep them in the house at all.

- Learn the art of savoring small amounts of food. And then reason like Jean: "Every bite I taste of something is going to taste the same so I don't feel psychologically deprived."

- If you begin to eat and feel that stopping will be difficult, throw out the food. Wasting food is better than overeating.

- Drink water or carbonated water for a feeling of fullness.

- Walk or exercise to dissipate anxiety.

- From the perspective of an objective observer or witness, visualize yourself stop eating.

- Repeat to yourself the affirmation, "I am not overeating."

- Use cognitive therapy on yourself to control food cravings like Diane, who says, "When I go to bakeries, I would love to buy more breads and things. I just don't. I think about what the consequences are going to be and that stops me."

- Follow a healthy diet with vegetables, fruits, whole grains, and legumes, low in sugar and fat. It may take several months, but you should experience fewer food cravings over time.

- Realize that food cravings come and go, so learn to go with the flow.

Food cravings may eventually burn themselves out. Linda tells us, "I realized I was going to have to pay for it if I ate a whole box of cookies. I might have to starve myself the next day. I think I just got sick of doing that, sick of the ups and downs, and realizing I wasn't really enjoying that box of cookies. The first few cookies were great but then after that, you can't taste them anymore."

Depression

Signs of depression are inability to enjoy yourself, difficulty concentrating, feelings of hopelessness, fatigue, insomnia or sleeping too much, increased or decreased appetite, and thoughts of death or suicide. If you are not able to function well because of depression, see a professional counselor.

Social eating

Social eating is tricky because you want to eat enough to feel part of the group and not feel deprived, but you don't want to eat so much that you're uncomfortable afterwards. Use your good judgment.

Restaurants:

• Before sitting down, check the menu to make sure there is something that will be appropriate for you to eat.

• If others are ordering alcoholic drinks and you prefer not to drink, order juice or a carbonated beverage so you will not feel left out.

• Avoid being excessively hungry when you go out to eat by having a snack beforehand. Deborah comments, "I don't starve before going to a restaurant. I normally eat a piece of fruit or drink water."

• Ask for salad dressing on the side. Order fish broiled with lemon juice rather than butter. Remember Jean's words: "When you go out to eat, you can eat whatever you want to eat because you have control over what you tell the waitress you want."

• If you are served a large portion, plan to take home what you do not want to finish. Or order appetizers as a main course. Phyllis tells us, "People will say, 'The portions are fantastic.' Well, you don't need that kind of portion. You don't need the big buffet that you can eat until they have to wheel you out. That's habit. It isn't necessary."

• If you crave a dessert high in fat and sugar, share it with someone else. Or order tea, coffee, or fruit instead. But maybe you are like Marilyn, who says, "It's not that I can't have dessert. I don't want it, so why bother eating something I'm not very interested in."

- Enjoy the conversation and service rather than focusing on the food.
- When possible, plan social activities that do not include eating out.

Parties:

- Eat a snack before you go, so you will not be voraciously hungry when you arrive.
- Stay clear of the food table.
- If the party is pot luck, bring a low fat main course. Choose foods that are low in fat.
- To take your mind off eating, mingle. Diane focuses on the people at parties rather than food: "You feel you are at a party, so you should eat. But you don't have to eat if you don't want to. I load my plate up with vegetables or whatever they have that is appropriate. Or I'll take a very small amount of something and make it last all night. But parties to me are more for socializing, getting together with friends. The food is not that important."

Holiday celebrations—Thanksgiving to New Year's:

- Freeze high sugar, high fat foods you receive as gifts. Or give them away.
- After the gathering, consider following Jean's example: "When we have Thanksgiving in our house, I will give all the food away, all the pies, anything sweet, but we keep the turkey."
- Remember to schedule in time to exercise. Deborah has learned, "At holiday times, I really stress the exercise. You have to balance it."

Work

Eating nutritious foods at work can be a challenge.

- Rather than eating cafeteria food, which usually is not low in fat, bring your own lunch to work. If there is not enough time in the morning to make your lunch, prepare it the evening before or purchase a healthy frozen meal to heat up in a microwave.

- Contribute food low in sugar and fat to the coffee room snacks.
- To relieve the stress of work, take a walk at lunchtime.

Home

Many people have a tendency to overeat when they are home alone. To change this habit, try the following:

- Choose to eat only in the kitchen or dining room. Then other rooms are not associated with eating. If you find yourself overeating, going into a food-free room is one way of helping yourself stop eating.

- If you are usually famished when you arrive home after work and tend to run directly to the refrigerator, eat a snack before leaving work. By the time you arrive home, you will not be as hungry.

- Take your mind off food by focusing on other activities, such as a long-postponed project, calling a friend, reading a book, doing handwork, or listening to music. Have a list ready of things to do.

- Plan to have one satisfying evening snack. Otherwise try to stay away from the kitchen.

Traveling

Traveling usually means eating out, and a variable schedule.

- Make every effort to eat nutritious foods. Try to follow a schedule for meals and snacks.

- Set aside time during the day to exercise and relax. Get a good night's sleep.

- Visualize yourself returning home still being able to fit into your clothes.

✦ *When are you most likely to overeat?*

IF YOU DO OVEREAT

If you do overeat, do not punish yourself. Remember the times you were able to avoid overeating. Tell yourself that this was an isolated event, separate from the past and the future. It was just a bump in the road and you will get another chance to challenge yourself.

Review the situation and ask yourself what caused you to overeat. How would you act differently the next time? Imagine a similar situation and visualize yourself using the skills you've learned to change your behavior.

Linda comments, "If there are occasions when I eat more than usual, I know I am going to go back to my usual eating habits the next day, so I don't make an issue of it." Deborah advises, "So you overdo it on a certain day. But the key is to say, 'Well, I blew that,' and to get up and get on with it. It balances over time."

✦ *Do you overeat? If so, how do you react afterwards?*

CHAPTER 6

TRANSITIONING TO LONG-TERM WEIGHT MAINTENANCE

Congratulations! You have taken off some weight and have decided to stabilize at your new healthier weight. Your goal is to keep it off. Allow a period of time to adjust to your lower weight and to learn to deal with feelings and thoughts that might sabotage your efforts to maintain your weight. To learn from your past experiences, review why you think you gained weight previously. Monitor your weight and keep yourself motivated. Continue to improve your self-esteem and body image, maintain your exercise program, choose nutritious foods, and prevent yourself from overeating.

ADJUSTING TO A NEW BODY WEIGHT

It may take several months to develop a new body image that is in keeping with your new weight and to learn how to balance the amount of food you eat with your physical activity.

A new body image

People who have lost weight may have a distorted body image, seeing themselves as heavier than they really are. Marilyn tells us, "It was a while before I realized I had to buy smaller clothes. It's probably when I started wearing clothes that fit that I noticed I weighed less." It is important to be able to 'see' your weight change so you can praise yourself for your accomplishment and feel good about it. This will reinforce the lifestyle changes you have made and keep you motivated.

Anxiety about food

You may be afraid that eating any 'extra' food will put on weight. Phyllis remembers, "You go through a period where you feel that if you eat one extra thing, you are going to blow up. It takes several months for you to feel comfortable and at ease with yourself. I think I'm beyond that now."

Getting enough exercise

Don't get out of the exercise habit. Nicole realized the importance of physical activity for weight management. She recalls, "It was constant testing out for maybe three to five months. Then I discovered that, if for any reason I can not get the exercise, I will go up a pound or two. I know myself now."

FEELINGS AND THOUGHTS CAN SABOTAGE WEIGHT MAINTENANCE

Be prepared for feelings and thoughts that prevent you from keeping the weight off. Examples are given here, but be aware of others unique to you.

Disappointment from unmet social expectations

Linda recalls, "Like a lot of women, I thought I'd be more attractive to men [after losing weight], that I'd feel more comfortable around people. That wasn't necessarily so." It may seem as if weight management is not worth the effort because you have not attained your social goals. If so, come up with more stable long-term motivations for wanting to maintain your weight, such as those on pages 5–6.

Discomfort in relationships

The people who are important in your life may be threatened by the changes that are taking place. The previously established balance of the relationship may be disrupted. It may seem easier to regain the weight and continue in the old familiar ways of relating rather than try to create new ways of communicating, which takes effort and involves risk.

Fear of failing

Anne comments, "If you don't have the extra weight anymore, there is always an underlying feeling of, 'Gosh, I'm going to fail.' And it's not because I'm fat. It might be because I'm not good enough at my job or because they really don't like me." Extra weight can be used as an excuse for 'failing.' When you were overweight, if something wasn't going your way, you might have accused others of being prejudice towards overweight people. Now, you may be afraid that if you 'fail' at life's work and social challenges, it may be because you don't have the necessary work or social skills. This might create stress and bring up new feelings that are difficult to cope with and you might regain weight in order to avoid them. If this fear comes up, develop your self-esteem.

Disdain for the image of your heavier self

Nicole observes, "There is a connection and a disconnection with that person, but the core of me is still the same." You want to detach from the image of your heavier self so you can move on to new territory, but you do not want to dislike that person because you are, in fact, still that same person inside, just a smaller version. Any negative feelings you have towards yourself at any point in your life will only promote low self-esteem and create the potential for overeating.

Fear of following in someone else's footsteps

Anne tells us, "Seeing my sister getting fat again seems like a foreshadowing of what might happen to me." It is not realistic to think that because someone else regained weight, you will too. You are your own person.

Stress from problems kept on the back burner

When you are focused on weight management, it's easy to ignore other important issues. When the weight is lost, you may need to face those problems that have been put on the back burner. To deal with the stress, apply stress reduction techniques, join a support group, or see a professional counselor.

Uncomfortable feelings for victims of sexual abuse

When women who have been sexually abused begin to feel attractive, uncomfortable feelings may surface. If these painful feelings are not dealt with, usually with professional assistance, the individual may overeat to regain the weight as a way of avoiding these feelings.

✦ *Are there reasons why you might not want to be at a lower weight?*

REVIEW WHY YOU GAINED WEIGHT IN THE PAST

Just because you gained weight in the past doesn't mean you will this time because this is a different point in your life. But reviewing your past can give you insight to help you keep the weight off. Perhaps you recognize these reasons for gaining weight:

Louise: "It was kind of insidious how it crept up without my noticing it right away. I was more of a snacker. I was home and I didn't have the activity of the children being home. I was having lunch with my friends, doing more eating. I never was an exerciser, just some walking. I had to go to work and I was depressed so I took it out on food. I would look in the mirror and eat more. It was definitely a snowball effect." *Reasons for weight gain: excessive snacking, low physical activity, depression.*

Joseph: "I would eat, sit, read, go to class. I could get a lot of food cheap. I had nothing to do at home after work but eat." *Reasons for weight gain: low physical activity, too much food available, boredom.*

Ann: "I am not a binge eater, but I got fat by constant eating, although not a lot at one sitting." *Reason for weight gain: excessive snacking.*

Sarah: "When I moved to Washington, I was in a car a lot." *Reason for weight gain: low physical activity because of a life event change.*

Phyllis: "I put weight on in my mid-forties, but not dramatically. I inched up. I was not thinking about it. Then, when my husband got sick, I shot up to 170 and I didn't care." *Reasons for weight gain: adjusting to gradual weight gain, stress from family illness.*

Nicole: "I was in a depressing living situation. My weight went up over several years. I was in a new place with a small child. I reverted to eating." *Reasons for weight gain: adjusting to gradual weight gain, depression.*

✦ *Why did you gain weight in the past?*

MONITORING YOUR WEIGHT FOR MAINTENANCE

Step 1 – Choose a method

After you have reached a healthier weight, it is critical that you regularly monitor your weight. If you regain, you will know sooner rather than later. You can then reevaluate your behavior to get back on track.

One easy way to monitor your weight is by the fit of your clothes. This method works well for Anne, who tells us, "I mostly monitor my weight through the way clothes fit. The clothes always fit so I am sure everything is okay. I get weighed at the doctor's office so I do have some basis for reality."

Marilyn says, "My clothes are probably my best point of reference. If they start getting snug, then I start getting worried. I get on the scale and see where I am. Otherwise, I don't really weigh myself often, maybe once a month or in the doctor's office."

If you feel that your clothes are getting snug, the idea of weighing yourself may make you anxious. To lessen the anxiety, first get back on track, and when your clothes fit again, weigh yourself. By then, you will probably be back where you want and you will have avoided the anxiety of a higher number on the scale staring you in the face.

An additional way to monitor your weight is to weigh yourself every few weeks, at least until you are confident that you will be able to keep off the weight you've lost long-term. Now you are looking for a trend of increasing weight, a warning sign that will motivate you to get back on track right away. Weighing yourself during weight maintenance should not be as anxiety provoking as when you were losing weight because it won't take you a long time to lose a few pounds.

✦ *Now that you want to keep your weight stable, how do you plan to monitor your weight?*

Step 2 – Establish a weight range

For example, a weight range for a weight of 150 pounds might be 147 to 153. "I give myself a three pound maximum gain," says Edward. "I know I can reverse that in a short time." If the weight range you choose is too difficult to maintain, then adjust it upward to one that is less stressful to maintain.

✦ *What is your weight range?*

Step 3 – Create a plan to get back on track

If you have exceeded your upper limit, have a plan in mind for taking off the extra weight. Here are a few examples:

Anne: "I would think about my eating patterns to see if I crept into a pattern I hadn't noticed. If I were eating a lot more fat in my diet, I would try to cut it out. I would make sure that I exercised."

Marilyn: "I would cut out non-meal foods such as snack foods that I eat with my kids. Otherwise, I would probably have to step up my exercise. I would eat a little less at dinner."

✦ *If you were to regain some weight, how would you get back on track?*

KEEPING UP YOUR MOTIVATION

When you were losing the weight, you probably received compliments and encouragement from family and friends, but now that you have achieved a healthier weight and stabilized, the positive feedback may have disappeared. You will need to motivate yourself. You can do this by reminding yourself of the benefits you reap from being at a healthier weight. Your self-motivation may be similar to these:

Anne: "I feel healthier. I have less trouble with my knees. It's easier to buy clothes. It's easier to move around. I think I look better." *Self-motivation: improved health, easier to find clothes that fit, feeling good about self.*

Patricia: "I feel better. I like to buy clothes and I like to wear clothes." *Self-motivation: improved health, easier to find clothes that fit.*

Marilyn: "Especially having little kids, I can do things with them I couldn't do before, like sitting in a rocking chair. I think it's more fun. I don't have to worry about health factors because what I am doing right now I perceive to be healthy. I had gestational diabetes, so if I gained weight, I could have some health complications. I think that's a pretty good motivation to keep the weight off." *Self-motivation: able to expand enjoyable activities, minimal worries about health.*

Sarah: "I feel better when I don't eat a lot of fat. I know I can eat enough and still feel full, so it isn't punitive. Now I'm being good to myself." *Self-motivation: improved health, way to treat self well.*

Edward: "I never liked the fact that clothes were uncomfortable, that it was a struggle to get my shoes on. It's nice to be able to pull on my pants standing on one foot. It's nice to be making more holes in my belts rather than buying bigger belts. My blood pressure has dropped." *Self-motivation: feeling more comfortable physically, improved health.*

Phyllis: "Maintaining the weight is a way of keeping healthy. It's a way of keeping young. It's a way of keeping yourself productive. I am much healthier. I can walk up to the fourth floor. I could not have done that before. I am 65. I am in good health and I want to stay this way. At a certain point, vanity took over. I like the way I look. I like the way I feel." *Self-motivation: able to be more active, improved health, feeling good about self.*

✦ *How do you benefit from being at a healthier weight?*

A CONTINUAL LEARNING PROCESS

For weight maintenance, continue to apply the four approaches and techniques used for weight loss, but now the time span is long-term.

Feeling good about yourself

- Maintain vigilant watch to be sure you hold onto your new improved self-image.

- Have a mission in life. A purpose outside of yourself will make you feel good about yourself and also distract you from food. For example, your mission might be to teach high school students, raise a well-adjusted family, or own a business. It may take time to figure this out but it is important to do.

- Develop new interests and hobbies. They will help you improve your self-esteem by getting to know yourself better and can also open up opportunities for social relationships.

Maintaining an exercise program

- Continue to choose a variety of activities you enjoy for each season of the year.

- Keep up-to-date on research findings about exercise by reading newspapers, books, and magazines. The Nutrition Counseling and Education Services, listed under Resources at the end of this book, publishes a catalogue with descriptions of books and videos on exercise.

Choosing nutritious foods

- Continue to choose nutritious foods and try new ones.

- Learn ways to prepare them to your liking. Taking cooking classes is one way to learn how to prepare healthy foods. But remember, cooking well is an art and a science that takes time to learn.

Preventing overeating

- Continue to become more aware of your thoughts and feelings. This is a life-long, growth promoting process that is key to weight management.

- Gain experience in problem-solving techniques because there will always be problems to solve. Seek help from a support system as needed.

- Learn to cope with changing life situations that can be stressful. Try to figure out what you can and cannot change in your life. Phyllis had to do this: "My gaining weight is not going to help my husband's medical condition. I can't change that. The only thing I have control over is me, and I'm going to maintain that control. This is something that every one can do. You have to have that mindset."

• Take time out to enjoy yourself to relieve stress and anxiety. Bear in mind that what you enjoy doing may change over time as your interests and focus shift.

• Enhance your social relationships. Appreciate social relationships that offer such benefits as conversation, caring, and mutual respect. Learn how to constructively handle feelings of rejection, criticism, and anger that both you and the other person might experience in a relationship. When conflict arises, listen and communicate so you can create a win-win situation that benefits all involved.

• Expand your life by doing volunteer work in your community.

Long-term weight management is an ongoing process that gets easier and for which the rewards become greater with time. The longer you maintain your weight, the better your chances are for keeping it off. Each day counts because those days add up to weeks, months, and years in which you will have maintained your weight.

WE'D LIKE TO HEAR FROM YOU. SEND YOUR COMMENTS TO FINDING YOUR WAY TO A HEALTHIER WEIGHT, GENERAL CLINICAL RESEARCH CENTER, BOX 831, NEW ENGLAND MEDICAL CENTER, 750 WASHINGTON STREET, BOSTON, MASSACHUSETTS 02111.

GUIDELINES FOR HEALTHY WEIGHTS

Height [1]		Weight [2]
5 ft.	0 in.	97–128 lbs.
5	1	101–132
5	2	104–137
5	3	107–141
5	4	111–146
5	5	114–150
5	6	118–155
5	7	121–160
5	8	125–164
5	9	129–169
5	10	132–174
5	11	136–179
6	0	140–184
6	1	144–189
6	2	148–195
6	3	152–200
6	4	156–205
6	5	160–211
6	6	164–216

[1] Without shoes. [2] Without clothes. The higher weights apply to people, such as many men, who have more muscle and bone. Source: 1990 and 1995 Dietary Guidelines for Americans.

APPENDIX B

20% AND 30% FAT DIETS

A 20% / 30% fat diet means that 20% / 30% of the total calories in the diet comes from fat. To translate this into fat grams in the diet, the total calories is multiplied by 20% and 30% and this value is divided by 9, which is the number of calories per gram of fat. (For example, 2000 total calories multiplied by 0.3 equals 600 calories from fat. 600 calories divided by 9 calories per gram of fat equals 67 grams of fat.) See the chart below for fat grams in 20% and 30% fat diets at various calorie levels.

If you want to follow a 20% or a 30% fat diet to maintain (or lose) weight, follow these steps:

1) **Determine the number of calories you need to maintain your weight.** The total calories you need to maintain your weight depends on several factors, so there is no simple calculation for caloric requirements. You can estimate the calories you need to maintain your weight by first writing down the foods and portion sizes you eat on a typical day, when necessary using measuring cups and spoons to measure portion sizes, and then looking up the calories in these foods using the Food Table on page 60, food labels, and a calorie counter booklet. (When aiming to lose weight at the rate of one-half to one pound per week, decrease the daily calorie level you need to maintain your weight by 250 to 500 calories.)

2) Look up in the chart below the number of grams of fat for a 20% or 30% fat diet at that calorie level. Your goal would be to limit the fat grams you eat daily to this number.

3) Be aware of the number of fat grams you eat daily. Keep a record of the food you eat and check the number of fat grams in the Food Table, on food labels, and in a fat gram counter booklet.

For example, if you estimated that you typically ate 2000 calories daily and if you decided you wanted to follow a 30% or less fat diet, you would try to eat fewer than 67 grams of fat daily. If you had for breakfast 1 orange (0 grams of fat), 1/2 cup of oatmeal (1 gram of fat), 1 cup of 1% milk (3 grams of fat), 1 slice of whole wheat bread (1 gram of fat), and 2 teaspoons of peanut butter (5 grams of fat), you would have had 10 grams of fat for breakfast and would try to limit the fat grams you ate for the rest of the day to 57 grams.

Calories	20% FAT DIET Grams of Fat	30% FAT DIET Grams of Fat
1400	31	47
1600	36	53
1800	40	60
2000	44	67
2200	49	73
2400	53	80
2600	58	87
2800	62	93
3000	67	100

APPENDIX C

EXAMPLES OF MEALS

Below are examples of basic breakfasts (whole grain, food source of protein, fruit) and lunches/dinners (whole grain, food source of protein, vegetable). Meals need to be seasoned to the individual's taste.

BREAKFASTS	LUNCHES/DINNERS
whole grain: **food source of protein:** **fruit:**	**whole grain:** **food source of protein:** **vegetable:**
whole wheat bread egg orange	brown rice black beans green beans
shredded wheat milk banana	whole wheat bread tuna fish dark green salad
multi-grain cooked cereal soy yogurt raisins	buckwheat tofu broccoli, carrots
oatmeal yogurt blueberries	whole wheat pasta ground meat in tomato sauce cauliflower
whole wheat bread soy cheese apple	oat groats chickpeas acorn squash
whole wheat bread cottage cheese pineapple	soup: barley chicken turnip, onion
ready-to-eat whole wheat cereal soy milk strawberries	millet adzuki beans kale

FOOD TABLE

Reason for including the Food Table: The basic nutrition message of this book is to choose to eat tasty, nutritious foods that are low in fat, eating when physiologically hungry, stopping when full, and to aim to distribute the major nutrients - carbohydrate, protein, fat, and fiber—among three meals. Weight loss should follow for the reasons on page 35. This message is presented in the text in concepts rather than using structured meal plans and nutritional food values because some readers will not like to work with numbers. The Food Table is included here for those individuals who would prefer to plan their meals using nutritional food values.

Overview of Food Table: The subheadings **Dairy, Fruits, Grains, Legumes, Meats, Nuts, Oils, Seeds, Vegetables, and Other** are the same as those for the food lists on pages 27–30. For each food item, the portion size, food energy in units of calories, and the protein, carbohydrate, and fat in units of grams are given.

Food items: The food items listed are the same as those in the food lists on pages 27–30. They were chosen because they are representative of nutritious foods people are generally familiar with and as a group provide enough variety to make a healthy diet interesting.

Portion sizes: The portion sizes for food items were chosen for various reasons. The portion sizes for the **Nuts, Oils,** and **Seeds** were chosen for convenience in counting fat grams which is explained in Appendix B. The half-cup portion sizes for the **Vegetables** and **Fruits** are standard but three to five servings of vegetables and two to four servings of fruits daily make up an important part of a healthy diet. Two to three one-cup portion sizes of low fat milk and/or yogurt from the **Dairy** group provide significant calcium each day to help lessen bone loss associated with aging. The portion sizes for **Grains, Legumes,** and **Meats** would most likely be satisfying for an individual of smaller physique who is about five feet in height. However, a person of larger physique who is about six feet in height might prefer portion sizes two to three times these amounts.

Nutritional food values for calories and fat in grams per portion size: These food values are needed to calculate 20% / 30% fat diets as referred to on pages 32–33 and explained in *Appendix B*.

Nutritional food values for protein, carbohydrate, and fiber in grams per portion size: These were included to show that certain foods listed on page 27–30 are in fact better sources of these nutrients relative to other sources. This information is useful when aiming to distribute the major nutrients in foods among three meals as referred to on pages 34–35.

How to use the Food Table to plan a meal: If you were planning to eat one of the meals in Appendix C, for example, brown rice (a whole grain), black beans (a food source of protein), and green beans (a vegetable), you would learn from looking up the food values of the major nutrients in these foods in the Food Table that:

- the protein in the meal would come mainly from the black beans (8 grams per 1/2 cup) but also in smaller amounts from the brown rice (2 grams per 1/2 cup) and green beans (1 gram per 1/2 cup)
- the carbohydrate in the meal would come mainly from the brown rice (23 grams) and black beans (20 grams) but also in a smaller amount from the green beans (5 grams)
- the fiber would come mainly from the black beans (8 grams) but also in smaller amounts from the brown rice (2 grams) and green beans (1 gram)
- the total fat content from the brown rice (1 gram), black beans (less than 0.5 grams), and green beans (less than 0.5 grams) was low, making it acceptable to add to the meal measured amounts of fat (as determined using the tool of counting fat grams explained in Appendix B) in the form of tasty sauces, nuts, or seeds.

Measurement Equivalents

Volume
3 teaspoons = 1 tablespoon
2 tablespoons = 1 fluid ounce
8 fluid ounces = 1 cup

Weight
28 grams = 1 ounce
16 ounces = 1 pound

Sources of nutritional food values: Food Processor 6.0, ESHA Research, Salem, Oregon, unless otherwise noted. The pound sign (#) indicates food values from *Bowes and Church's Food Values of Portions Commonly Used*, revised by Jean AT Pennington, PhD,RD, Lippincott, New York, 1994.
Food values are rounded off to the nearest gram. The dot in place of a number for a food value indicates less than 0.5 grams, an insignificant amount.

FOOD ITEM, PORTION	Food Energy CALORIES	Protein GRAMS	Carbo-hydrate GRAMS	Fat GRAMS	Fiber GRAMS
DAIRY					
Cheese, cottage, 1% fat, 1/2 cup	82	14	3	1	0
Cheese, ricotta, part-skim, 2 ounces	78	6	3	4	0
Milk, 1% fat, 1 cup	102	8	12	3	0
Yogurt, low fat, 1 cup	155	13	17	3	0
FRUITS					
Apple, with peel, 1 medium	81	•	21	•	3
Apricots, dried halves, 10	83	1	22	•	3
Banana, 1 medium	105	1	28	1	2
Blackberries, 1/2 cup	38	1	9	•	3
Blueberries, 1/2 cup	41	•	10	•	2
Cantaloupe, cubes, 1 cup	56	1	13	•	1
Cherries, 10	49	1	11	1	1
Cranberries, raw, 1/2 cup	23	•	6	•	1
Dates, whole, 3	68	•	18	•	2
Figs, dried, 2	95	1	24	•	3
Grapefruit, 1/2 medium	37	1	9	•	2

Food Item, Portion	Food Energy CALORIES	Protein GRAMS	Carbo-hydrate GRAMS	Fat GRAMS	Fiber GRAMS
Grapes, Thompson, 1/2 cup	57	1	14	•	•
Nectarine, 1 medium	67	1	16	1	2
Orange, 1 medium	62	1	16	•	2
Peach, peeled, 1 medium	37	1	10	•	2
Pear, 1 medium	98	1	25	1	4
Pineapple, chunks, 1/2 cup	38	•	10	•	1
Plum, 2 medium	72	1	17	1	3
Prunes, 3	60	1	16	•	2
Raisins, 1/4 cup	109	1	29	•	1
Raspberries, 1/2 cup	30	1	7	•	2
Strawberries, whole, 1 cup	43	1	10	1	2

GRAINS

Food Item, Portion	Food Energy CALORIES	Protein GRAMS	Carbo-hydrate GRAMS	Fat GRAMS	Fiber GRAMS
Barley, whole, cooked, 1/2 cup	135	4	30	1	7
Barley, pearl, 1/2 cup	97	2	22	•	4
Bread, whole wheat, 1 slice	86	3	16	1	2
Buckwheat, groats, cooked, 1/2 cup	91	3	20	1	2
Bulgur, cooked, 1/2 cup	76	3	17	•	4
Cereal, cooked, multigrain, 1/2 cup	100	3	20	1	2
Cereal, ready-to-eat, wheat, 1 cup	101	3	23	•	3
Couscous, cooked, 1/2 cup	100	3	21	•	1
Millet, cooked, 1/2 cup	143	4	28	1	2
Oatmeal, cooked, 1/2 cup	73	3	13	1	2
Oat groats, cooked, 1/2 cup	121	5	21	2	3
Pasta, whole wheat, cooked, 1/2 cup	87	4	19	•	3
Rice, brown, cooked, 1/2 cup	110	2	23	1	2
Whole wheat berries, cooked, 1/2 cup	42	2	10	•	2

LEGUMES

Food Item, Portion	Food Energy CALORIES	Protein GRAMS	Carbo-hydrate GRAMS	Fat GRAMS	Fiber GRAMS
Adzuki beans, cooked, 1/2 cup	147	9	29	•	7
Black beans, cooked, 1/2 cup	114	8	20	•	8
Chickpeas, cooked, 1/2 cup	135	7	23	2	4
Kidney beans, cooked, 1/2 cup	113	8	20	•	7

Food Item, Portion	Food Energy CALORIES	Protein GRAMS	Carbo-hydrate GRAMS	Fat GRAMS	Fiber GRAMS
Lentils, cooked, 1/2 cup	115	9	20	•	5
Lima beans, cooked, 1/2 cup	108	7	20	•	7
Navy beans, cooked, 1/2 cup	129	8	24	1	8
Pinto beans, cooked, 1/2 cup	117	7	22	•	7

MEATS

Food Item, Portion	Food Energy CALORIES	Protein GRAMS	Carbo-hydrate GRAMS	Fat GRAMS	Fiber GRAMS
Beef, lean, ground, broiled, 2 ounces	166	17	0	10	0
Chicken, light meat, roasted, 2 ounces	112	17	0	4	0
Cod, baked, 2 ounces	58	13	0	•	0
Egg, 1 large	78	6	1	5	0
Egg, substitute, 1/4 cup	53	8	•	2	0
Flounder, baked, 2 ounces	64	13	0	1	0
Haddock, broiled, 2 ounces	64	14	0	1	0
Halibut, broiled, 2 ounces	79	15	0	2	0
Salmon, cooked, 2 ounces	103	14	0	5	0
Tuna, white, canned in water, 2 ounces	77	15	0	1	0
Turkey, light meat, roasted, 2 ounces	79	17	0	1	0

NUTS

Food Item, Portion	Food Energy CALORIES	Protein GRAMS	Carbo-hydrate GRAMS	Fat GRAMS	Fiber GRAMS
Almond butter, 2 teaspoons	67	2	2	6	1
Almonds, 6 nuts	42	1	1	4	•
Almonds, ground, 4 teaspoons	46	2	1	4	1
Cashew butter, 2 teaspoons	62	2	3	6	•
Cashews, 6 nuts	54	2	3	5	•
Macadamia, 3 nuts	51	1	1	5	•
Walnuts, ground, 1 teaspoons	48	1	1	5	•
Walnuts, halves, 5 halves	65	1	2	6	•

OILS

Food Item, Portion	Food Energy CALORIES	Protein GRAMS	Carbo-hydrate GRAMS	Fat GRAMS	Fiber GRAMS
Canola, 1 teaspoon	40	0	0	5	0
Corn, 1 teaspoon	40	0	0	5	0
Olive, 1 teaspoon	40	0	0	5	0
Peanut, 1 teaspoon	40	0	0	5	0

Food Item, Portion	Food Energy CALORIES	Protein GRAMS	Carbo-hydrate GRAMS	Fat GRAMS	Fiber GRAMS
Sesame, 1 teaspoon	40	0	0	5	0
Safflower, 1 teaspoon	40	0	0	5	0

SEEDS

Food Item, Portion	Food Energy	Protein	Carbo-hydrate	Fat	Fiber
Pumpkin, 47 seeds	47	2	2	4	•
Sesame butter (tahini), 2 teaspoons	61	2	2	6	1
Sesame, hulled, 1 tablespoon	52	2	2	4	1
Sunflower, 1 tablespoon	51	2	2	4	1

VEGETABLES

Food Item, Portion	Food Energy	Protein	Carbo-hydrate	Fat	Fiber
Acorn squash, cooked, 1/2 cup	68	1	18	•	5
Alfalfa sprouts, 1/2 cup	5	1	1	•	•
Asparagus, 1/2 cup	22	2	4	•	2
Bean sprouts, mung, raw, 1/2 cup	16	2	3	•	1
Beets, cooked, diced, 1/2 cup	37	1	8	•	1
Broccoli, cooked, pieces, 1/2 cup	22	2	4	•	2
Brussel sprouts, cooked, 1/2 cup	30	2	7	•	4
Butternut squash, cooked, 1/2 cup	49	1	13	•	3
Cabbage, raw, shredded, 1/2 cup	9	1	2	•	1
Carrots, sliced, cooked, 1/2 cup	35	1	8	•	2
Cauliflower, cooked, 1/2 cup	14	1	3	•	1
Celery, 1 stalk	6	•	1	•	1
Collards, cooked, 1/2 cup	17	1	4	•	1
Corn, cooked, 1/2 cup	66	2	17	•	2
Eggplant, cubed, cooked, 1/2 cup	14	•	3	•	1
Green beans, cooked, 1/2 cup	22	1	5	•	1
Greens, dark, mixed, 1 cup	9	1	2	•	1
Kale, cooked, 1/2 cup	21	1	4	•	1
Mushrooms, raw, 1/2 cup	2	•	•	•	•
Onion, 1 medium	42	1	10	•	2
Peas, cooked, 1/2 cup	67	4	13	•	2
Pepper, 1 medium	20	1	5	•	1
Pumpkin, cooked, 1/2 cup	25	1	6	•	1

Food Item, Portion	Food Energy CALORIES	Protein GRAMS	Carbo-hydrate GRAMS	Fat GRAMS	Fiber GRAMS
Rhubarb, diced, 1/2 cup	13	1	3	•	1
Spinach, raw, 1 cup	12	2	2	•	2
Squash, summer, cooked, 1/2 cup	18	1	4	•	1
Squash, winter, slices, cooked, 1/2 cup	47	1	11	1	3
Sweet potato, peeled, mashed, 1/2 cup	103	2	24	•	3
Tomato, raw, 1 medium	25	1	6	•	1
Turnips, cubes, cooked, 1/2 cup	14	1	4	•	2
Yam, baked, peeled, mashed, 1/2 cup	103	2	24	•	3
Zucchini squash, 1/2 cup	14	1	4	•	1

OTHER

Food Item, Portion	Food Energy CALORIES	Protein GRAMS	Carbo-hydrate GRAMS	Fat GRAMS	Fiber GRAMS
Avocado, mashed, 2 tablespoons	46	1	2	4	1
Hummus, 3 tablespoons	78	2	9	4	2
Mayonnaise, 1 teaspoon	33	•	•	4	0
Mayonnaise, light, 1 tablespoon	36	•	3	3	0
Olives, green, 10	45	1	1	5	•
Peanut butter, 2 teaspoons	63	3	2	5	1
Peanuts, 8 nuts	55	2	2	5	1
Soy milk, 1 cup	79	7	4	5	3
Tofu, raw, regular, 4 ounces	86	9	2	5	1

BIBLIOGRAPHY

✦ *Some of these books may be available in your public library*

Johnna Albi and Catherine Walthers, GREENS, GLORIOUS GREENS, St. Martin's Press: New York, 1996.

Bob Anderson, STRETCHING, Shelter: Bolinas, California, 1980.

Nathaniel Branden, SIX PILLARS OF SELF-ESTEEM, Bantam: New York, 1994.

Mark Bricklin and Linda Konner, YOUR PERFECT WEIGHT, Rodale: Emmaus, Pennsylvania, 1995.

Jane Brody, JANE BRODY'S GOOD FOOD BOOK, Bantam: New York, 1987.

Kelly D. Brownell, THE LEARN PROGRAM FOR WEIGHT CONTROL, The Learn Education Center: Dallas, 1994.

Kelly D. Brownell and J. Rodin, THE WEIGHT MAINTENANCE SURVIVAL GUIDE, Brownell and Hager: Dallas, 1990.

David D. Burns, FEELING GOOD: THE NEW MOOD THERAPY, Avon: New York, 1992.

Robert H. Colvin and Susan C. Olson, KEEPING IT OFF, Gilliland: Arkansas City, Kansas, 1989.

Martha Davis, Elizabeth Robbins Eshelman and Matthew McKay, THE RELAXATION AND STRESS REDUCTION WORKBOOK, New Harbinger: Oakland, California, 1988.

Albert Ellis and Robert A. Harper, A NEW GUIDE TO RATIONAL

LIVING, Prentice-Hall: Englewood Cliffs, New Jersey, 1975.

James M. Ferguson, HABITS, NOT DIETS, Bull, Palo Alto, 1988.

Anne M. Fletcher, THIN FOR LIFE, Chapters: Shelburne, Vermont, 1994.

John P. Foreyt and G. Kenneth Goodrick, LIVING WITHOUT DIETING, Harrison Publishing: Houston, 1992.

Daniel Goleman, EMOTIONAL INTELLIGENCE: WHY IT CAN MATTER MORE THAN IQ, Bantam: New York, 1995.

Michael Hamilton, Ronette L. Kolotkin, Diane F. Cogburn, and D.T. Moore, THE DUKE UNIVERSITY MEDICAL CENTER BOOK OF DIET AND FITNESS, Fawcett Columbine: New York, 1990.

Louise Hart, ON THE WINGS OF SELF-ESTEEM, Celestial Arts: Berkeley, 1994.

Jane R. Hirschman and Carol H. Munter, OVERCOMING OVEREATING, Fawcett Columbine: New York, 1989.

Agnes Huber, EATING FOR GOOD HEALTH AND PLEASURE, Vantage: New York, 1996.

Michelle Joy Levine, I WISH I WERE THIN, I WISH I WERE FAT, Ingham: LeVergne, Tennesse, 1997.

Barbara McFarland and Tyeis Baker-Baumann, SHAME AND BODY IMAGE, Health Communications: Deerfield Beach, Florida, 1990.

Laurel Mellin, THE SOLUTION: 6 WINNING WAYS TO PERMANENT WEIGHT LOSS, Harper Collins: New York, 1997.

Joyce D. Nash, NEW MAXIMIZE YOUR BODY POTENTIAL: LIFETIME SKILLS FOR WEIGHT MANAGEMENT, Bull: Palo Alto, 1996.

Joyce D. Nash, NOW THAT YOU'VE LOST IT: HOW TO MAINTAIN YOUR BEST WEIGHT, Bull: Palo Alto, 1992. *[This book includes an excellent discussion of the use of cognitive therapy in weight management.]*

Annette B. Natow and Jo-Ann Heslin, THE FAT COUNTER, Pocket Books: New York, 1993.

Miriam E. Nelson, STRONG WOMEN STAY THIN, Bantam: New York, 1998.

Linda Omichinski, YOU COUNT, CALORIES DON'T, Tamos Books: Winnipeg, Manitoba, Canada, 1992.

Susie Orbach, FAT IS A FEMINIST ISSUE II: A PROGRAM TO CONQUER COMPULSIVE OVEREATING, Berkley Books: New York, 1982.

Judith Rodin, BODY TRAPS, William Morrow: New York, 1992.

Irma S. Rombauer and Marion R. Becker, JOY OF COOKING, Nal-Dutton: New York, 1997.

Joanne Saltzman, AMAZING GRAINS, HJ Kramer: Tiburon, CA, 1990.

Joanne Saltzman, ROMANCING THE BEAN, HJ Kramer: Tiburon, CA, 1993.

Michael Samuels, HEALING WITH THE MIND'S EYE: A GUIDE FOR USING IMAGERY AND VISIONS FOR PERSONAL GROWTH AND HEALING, Summit: New York, 1990.

Lorna Sass, COMPLETE VEGETARIAN KITCHEN, Hearst: N.Y., 1992.

Lorna Sass, SHORT-CUT VEGETARIAN: GREAT TASTE IN NO TIME, Greenwillow: New York, 1997.

Virginia Satir, SELF-ESTEEM, Celestial Arts: Berkeley, 1995.

Evelyn Tribole and Elyse Resch, INTUITIVE EATING, St. Martin's Press: New York, 1995.

1995 US Dietary Guidelines for Americans, Superintendent of Documents, 202-512-1800

Doreen L. Virtue, THE YO-YO SYNDROME DIET, Harper and Row: New York, 1989.

SELECTED REFERENCES

Abernathy, R.P., and Black, D.R. (1996). Healthy body weights: an alternative perspective. *American Journal of Clinical Nutrition*, 63, 448S-451S.

Clark, M.M. (1996). Counseling strategies for obese patients. *American Journal of Preventive Medicine*, 12, 266-270.

Committee to Develop Criteria for Evaluating the Outcomes of Approaches to Prevent and Treat Obesity (1995). Weighing the options: criteria for evaluating weight-management programs. *Obesity Research*, 3, 591-604.

Cowburn, G., Hillsdon, M., and Hankey, C.R. (1997). Obesity management by life-style strategies. *British Medical Bulletin*, 53, 389-408.

Flatt, J.P. (1995). McCollum Award Lecture, 1995: Diet, lifestyle, and weight maintenance. *American Journal of Clinical Nutrition*, 62, 820-36.

Goldstein, D.J. (1992). Beneficial health effects of modest weight loss. *International Journal of Obesity*, 16, 397-415.

Jebb, S.A. (1997). Aetiology of obesity. *British Medical Bulletin*, 53, 264-285.

Klem, M.L., Wing, R.R., McGuire, M.T., Seagle, H.M., and Hill, J.O. (1997). A descriptive study of individuals successful at long-term maintenance of substantial weight loss. *American Journal of Clinical Nutrition*, 66, 239-246.

Loro, A.D., and Orleans, C.S. (1981). Binge eating in obesity: preliminary findings and guidelines for behavioral analysis and treatment. *Addictive Behaviors*, 6, 155-166.

Marlatt, G.A., and Gordon, J.R. (1985). *Relapse Prevention: Maintenance Strategies in Addictive Behavior Change*, Guilford: New York.

Meisler, J.G., and St. Jeor, S. (1996). Summary and recommendations from the American Health Foundation's expert panel on healthy weight, *American Journal of Clinical Nutrition*, 63, 474S-477S.

Perri, M.G., Sears, S.F., and Clark, J.E. (1993). Strategies for improving maintenance of weight loss. *Diabetes Care*, 16, 200-209.

Ravussin, E., Fontvieille, A.M., Swinburn, B.A., and Bogardus, C. (1993). Risk factors for the development of obesity, *Annals of the New York Academy of Sciences*, 683, 141-150.

Read, N., French, S., and Cunningham, K. (1994). The role of the gut in regulating food intake in man. *Nutrition Reviews*, 52, 1-10.

Rolls, B.J. (1995). Carbohydrates, fats, and satiety. *American Journal of Clinical Nutrition*, 61, 960S-967S.

St. Jeor, S.T. (1993). The role of weight management in the health of women. *Journal of the American Dietetic Association*, 93, 1007-1012.

Turner, L.W., Want, M.Q., and Westerfield, R.C. (1995). Preventing relapse in weight control: a discussion of cognitive and behavioral strategies. *Psychological Reports*, 77, 651-656.

Wadden, T.A., Steen, S.N., Wingate, B.J., and Foster, G.D. (1996). Psychosocial consequences of weight reduction: how much weight loss is enough? *American Journal of Clinical Nutrition*, 63, 461S-465S.

Willett, W.C. (1994). Diet and health: What should we eat? *Science*, 264, 532-537.

RESOURCES

American Dietetic Association Consumer Hotline
☎(800) 366-1655

American Institute for Cancer Research
brochures and newsletter with recipes and research on diet and cancer
1759 R Street, NW, Washington, DC 20069   ☎(800) 843-8114

Eating Disorders Awareness and Prevention
603 Stewart Street, Suite 803, Seattle, WA 98101   ☎(206) 382-3587

National Association for the Advancement of Fat Acceptance
P.O. Box 188620, Sacramento, CA 95818   ☎(916) 558-6880

Nutrition Counseling and Education Services
mail order company for books on nutrition, cookbooks, exercise, and eating disorders
1904 East 123rd Street, Olathe, KS 66061
☎(800) 445-5653 or (913) 782-4385

The Weight Control Digest
P.O. Box 35328, Dept. 30, Dallas, Texas 75235–0328   ☎(817) 545-4500

WIN
Weight Control Information Network
for packet of brochures, readings, and annotated bibliography
1 Win Way, Bethesda, Maryland, 20892–3665
☎(800) WIN-8098
http://www.niddk.nih.gov/

INDEX

Beans
cooking 28
food lists 27–28,30
storage 28
Body image 18–19, 47–48

Caffeine 33
Carbohydrate, food sources 28
Changes, ways to make 10–13
Childhood associations
with food 9
Cooking techniques 31

Diet
and health 26–27
and weight management 35
definition 26
guidelines for 32
meal planning 34–35
Dieting experiences 8–9

Exercise
aerobics 21
strengthening 23
stretching 21

Fat in diet
and health 32–33
food sources 29
how to decrease 33
saturated 33
20%, 30% fat diets 33, 57
Fiber, food sources 30
Food cravings, and overeating ... 41
Fruits, list 28, 30
Fullness, feeling of 36–37

Grains, whole
cooking 29
definition 27
food lists 28, 30
storage 29

Herbs and spices 31
Hunger, feeling of 36–37

Legumes, food lists 27–28, 30

Monitoring
weight loss 7–8
weight maintenance 51–52

Motivations
  weight loss 4
  weight maintenance 52–53
Nuts
  list 29
  storage 29
Oils
  list 29
  storage 29
Overeating
  and boredom 40
  and depression 43
  and emotions 38
  and fatigue 40
  and food cravings 41–42
  and procrastination 40
  and social eating 43–44
  and stress 39–40
  and thoughts 39
  at home 45
  at work 44
  traveling 45

Physical activity
  and health 20–21
  and weight management .. 20–21
  other considerations 23–24
  overcoming resistance 24–26
  types of exercise 21–23

Preparing meals
  reducing stress 34–35
Problem solving 13
Protein, food sources 27
Seeds
  food list 29
  storage 29
Self-esteem 15–18

Shopping, food 34
Snacks, lists 37–38
Social eating
  holidays 44
  parties 44
  restaurants 43–44
  work 44–45
Stress, and overeating 39–40
Support 13–14

Taste of nutritious foods 31
Tofu
  cooking 28
  storage 28

Vegetables
  list 30
  preparing 31

Water, in diet 33
Weight gain, reasons for 50–51
Weight maintenance
  sabotaging 48–50